I0831053

Advance Praise for *Comfort Always*

"An inspirational medical memoir about the forgotten art of healing. *Comfort Always* will make you laugh, cry, and marvel at the resilience of families facing the crisis of their lives."

—**Sanjay Gupta, MD**,
CNN chief medical correspondent

"Extraordinary stories about one of the most demanding fields of medicine—and much wisdom."

—**Dr. Henry Marsh, CBE, FRCS,**
British neurosurgeon and bestselling author of *Do No Harm: Stories of Life, Death and Brain Surgery*

"*Comfort Always* is a marvelous picture of the life of a pediatric neurosurgeon, his patients, and their families. Written with insight and feeling, Dr. Cohen engages the reader's mind and heart, brilliantly melding the science of medicine with the art of healing."

—**Jerome Groopman, MD,**
Recanati professor of medicine at Harvard Medical School and bestselling author of *How Doctors Think*

"Among pediatric neurosurgeons, Dr. Alan R. Cohen is known as a master surgeon, an extraordinary teacher, and an international leader in our field. To his young patients though, Dr. Cohen is 'Big Al' or 'Elvis' because of his hilarious and legendary Elvis Presley impersonation performances together with his patients. *Comfort Always* shares incredible stories, mostly of children with brain tumors, and conveys Dr. Cohen's kindness, compassion, humility, and humor. This book will inspire readers, as Dr. Cohen's stories describing both medical miracles and tragedies are so engaging, and his humanity shines through each one of them."

—**David Sandberg, MD**,
emeritus professor and chief of pediatric
neurosurgery at McGovern Medical School and
bestselling author of *Brain and Heart: The Triumphs
and Struggles of a Pediatric Neurosurgeon*

"Stories about sick children are beyond compelling for reasons of shared humanity. Dr. Al Cohen's neurosurgical stories tap into primal joy, fear, loss, and triumphs that can only be told by a surgeon who operates on the brains of children. With authenticity and humility, one of the country's most prominent surgeons opens a world that few have the fortitude to tread."

—**Allan H. Ropper, MD**,
professor of neurology at Harvard Medical School,
associate editor of *The New England Journal of
Medicine*, and bestselling author of *Reaching Down
the Rabbit Hole and How the Brain Lost Its Mind*

"*Comfort Always* is riveting! The one and only 'Big Al' Cohen has cared for thousands of children with tumors of the brain or spinal cord over the course of his phenomenal career, and now—finally!—he has written about the experience of both the challenging operations and the often difficult decisions or conversations that must happen around these charged moments. Sprinkling each story with humor, history, and a deep reverence for his patients and their parents, Big Al allows us a glimpse into a lifetime of lifesaving, and the massive heart of a man who is a treasure in our field."

—**Jay Wellons, MD**,
professor of neurological surgery at Vanderbilt University and
author of *All That Moves Us: A Pediatric Neurosurgeon, His
Young Patients, and Their Stories of Grace and Resilience*

Comfort Always

Comfort Always

Healing in the Age of Technology

ALAN R. COHEN, MD

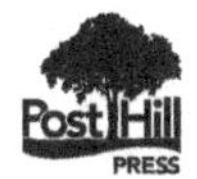

A POST HILL PRESS BOOK
ISBN: 979-8-89565-619-8
ISBN (eBook): 979-8-89565-620-4

Comfort Always:
Healing in the Age of Technology

Cover design by Jim Villaflores
Cover photo by John Tomsick

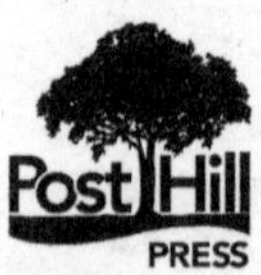

Post Hill Press
New York • Nashville
posthillpress.com

Published in the United States of America
1 2 3 4 5 6 7 8 9 10

For my courageous young patients,
From whom I have learned so much about the art of healing.

For the parents of my courageous young patients,
Thank you for the privilege of caring for those you hold most dearly.

"Our sorrows and wounds are healed only when we touch them with compassion."

—Buddha

CONTENTS

AUTHOR'S NOTE

The stories in this book are real. They have been generously shared by the families. The names have not been changed. Permission to use them was granted by the children or their parents.

Permission was also granted from the patient for use of her photograph on the book's cover. The picture was taken on September 16, 2005, when she was eleven years old in the pediatric intensive care unit, immediately following resection of a large posterior fossa brain tumor. Twenty years later, she is married with two young children of her own and working in a doggie day care center. She is tumor free.

PROLOGUE

"May I never forget that the patient is a fellow creature in pain. May I never consider him merely a vessel of disease."

Moses Maimonides (1135–1204)
Medieval philosopher, scholar, physician, rabbi

I am a neurosurgeon. More specifically, I am a pediatric neurosurgeon. I take care of children with surgical disorders of the nervous system. The work I do daily remains as fascinating to me today as it was when I began my career. The work is also unique—I didn't even know the specialty existed when I was in medical school. In this book, I hope to give the reader a glimpse of my world, with patient stories from my own practice, to elucidate the contributions of both technology and humanity in the art of healing.

My particular focus has been childhood brain tumors, and much of my attention is centered on the weighty tasks of attempting to preserve life and forestall death. The conversations I have with families are often profound and emotionally charged. At times, my job requires me to be the bearer of the worst news a parent could ever hope to hear: "I'm sorry to have to tell you this, but your child has a brain tumor." It is one of the hardest things I have ever had to do, and it doesn't get easier with time. To this day, I am haunted by those dreaded words in that simple sentence, knowing they will immediately turn the lives of the entire family upside down and remove any aspect of normalcy. The crushing sorrow brought on by that one sentence is unimaginable.

Despite the heartache of breaking bad news, and despite the many years of arduous training and the long hours at work, I feel lucky to be able to do what I do. Some of the happiest moments I've ever experienced have been helping a child and family navigate through a life-threatening illness. There is unparalleled joy in being able to tell a parent, "We were able to remove the tumor. It's benign, and your child is going to be okay." Even when the tumor is not benign, the outcomes in pediatric neurosurgery have improved dramatically since the subspecialty began almost a century ago. Huge advances have come about, even over the past decade. Novel, personalized treatments are often available, and more are on the immediate horizon, such that the diagnosis of a brain tumor is no longer a guaranteed death sentence. The future is getting brighter.

The path that brought me to my present position was unconventional. When I was a kid growing up in Poughkeepsie, New York, I remember watching a TV series called *Ben Casey*. It was a popular show that was centered on the daily life of a brilliant, intense neurosurgeon. It aired on ABC on Monday evenings from 1961 to 1966. During those five years, Ben Casey, played by the actor Vince Edwards, served as the talented, though often brusque, arrogant, and headstrong chief resident in neurosurgery at County General Hospital. He was sometimes cynical with his patients and often locked horns with the medical establishment.

I never even considered it unusual that Dr. Casey continued to remain chief resident for five consecutive years in the series without advancing in his career. I also never questioned the plot, which had him romantically involved with a woman—Jane Hancock, played by Stella Stevens—who had just awakened from a fifteen-year coma. I also remember multiple episodes in which Casey was called on to operate on patients with brain tumors.

The show was my first exposure to neurosurgery, and I was totally absorbed by the graphic medical drama. But I was pretty naïve in those days, and I really had no idea what a neurosurgeon did. I could never be like that, I thought. I don't have the right personality. I don't have the stamina. I was just a normal kid. Neurosurgeons were clearly crazy.

As far back as I can remember, I had always wanted to be a doctor. My dad was a major factor in that decision. He was an eye surgeon who was larger than life and had a profound influence on me. He was a self-made man who grew up in a poor neighborhood on the Lower East Side of New York City. With a combination of grit, determination, and hard work, he went on to become a revered physician and a pillar of our community. When I was a teenager, he used to bring me with him to the OR to observe him performing delicate microsurgery on the eye. It was beautiful to watch him work. He was a wonderful role model. I wanted to be like my dad. I wanted to be an ophthalmologist.

Gradually, it dawned on me that if I were to become an ophthalmologist, I would always be compared to my dad, and I would never be able to measure up to his standards. I would definitely need to find another specialty. Ophthalmology was out of the question. Not only was my dad a technical wizard in the OR, but he was also a very humble, modest man. I was surprised to learn that he had graduated first in his class in medical school, a fact that he had never shared with my mother. She only found out about it from an old classmate of his, years after they got married.

Sadly, that humility gene did not appear to be passed on to me. Humility is a trait that some people, like my dad, are born with. For others like me, it must be learned. And the learning curve is sometimes steep, as I will describe.

Poughkeepsie is a small town in upstate New York, where I attended a large public high school. I enjoyed my time there and formed many friendships, some of which have been lifelong. A good number of my classmates began working immediately after graduation. In what seemed like a miracle to me at the time, I was accepted to college at Harvard. I was overcome with a combination of excitement and fear. Immediately upon my arrival, I found myself in way over my head, surrounded by classmates—all of whom were geniuses. What was I doing there? It was a bumpy start, and I felt apprehensive and overwhelmed as I began my freshman year.

Things seemed to turn around for me during the second semester. I received a letter from Harvard stating that I was going to be awarded the Edwards Whitaker Scholarship in recognition of my "outstanding scholastic ability." Wow, maybe things weren't so bad after all. I proudly told my parents, and my mom promptly informed pretty much everyone she met in our hometown. For a time, I was walking around with an extra bounce in my step. I felt like a baseball player who had just made it to the majors.

My excitement was short-lived, though, dampened significantly several weeks later when I received official notification from Harvard: "You will be sent a check in the amount of $13.50 in the near future." Apparently, Harvard had a different view of my scholarship than I did. But I did learn a valuable lesson from the experience about humility and the benefit of having a modest view of one's own importance.

After college, I spent four years in medical school memorizing a lot of Latin terms and facts about anatomy and pathology and then set off for residency training in internal medicine. I chose medicine because I liked the challenges of physical diagnosis and particularly enjoyed the interactions with patients and families. But I soon became absorbed by the beauty of the human nervous system and the complexity of its associated disorders and promptly changed direction to begin my career in neurosurgery.

The human brain is an extraordinary structure, arguably the most complex object in the known universe. It is still shrouded in mystery despite centuries of thoughtful research. With a weight of about three pounds, it is made up of 75 percent water and has the texture of jelly. The brain is estimated to contain about one hundred billion neurons (nerve cells), perhaps about half as many stars as there are in the Milky Way Galaxy. These neurons and their trillions of synapses (connections) are responsible for our consciousness, intelligence, and all aspects of our humanity.

Years later, when I was chief resident in neurosurgery at the New York University Medical Center, there was a framed photograph of Vince Edwards that hung on the wall of my office. It had been placed there years earlier by one of the former chief residents. It was signed by Edwards and carried the inscription, "To Joe Ransohoff, the real Ben Casey." Ransohoff, my mentor and department chairman, had served as medical adviser to the show. He was a gruff, no-nonsense, gifted neurosurgeon. It was easy for me to see how he had helped morph the TV character in his own image (though unlike Ben Casey, Ransohoff was adored by all his patients and trainees).

Even today, some consider the stereotypical neurosurgeon to be an arrogant, egotistical modern version of Ben Casey. And, for sure, there are still some holdovers from the old days. But they are the exception.

Neurosurgery is perhaps the ultimate violation of an individual's privacy. While it does require a certain amount of self-confidence to operate on the brain of another living human being, confidence is not the same as arrogance. Confidence is quiet. Arrogance is loud.

This is a book about the art of medicine in the age of modern technology. It is an account of lessons I have learned caring for patients in a career spanning four decades. I have attempted to showcase some of the remarkable scientific advances that have enabled physicians to combat disease, relieve suffering, and, in some cases, prolong life. But I have also emphasized the forgotten nontechnical factors important in the art of healing. My hope is that this message will resonate with a wide range of general readers, including those who have dealt personally with serious illness or have helped family members or friends manage the complexities of a dangerous disease.

Brain tumors, my particular focus, are the most common solid tumors in children. They have now earned the dubious distinction of being the leading cause of cancer death in this age group. Tumors of the central nervous system (CNS) comprise 20 percent of childhood cancers, making them second only to leukemia in frequency. Great strides have been made in the treatment of childhood leukemia over the past fifty years, and the five-year survival rate for acute lymphoblastic leukemia (ALL), the most common form of childhood leukemia, is now 90 percent. While the prognosis for children with brain tumors has improved across the board, it has lagged behind the success achieved in the treatment of leukemia. The survival rate for children with several types of malignant pediatric brain tumors has not improved significantly, and treatments can be associated with long-term toxicities.

Luckily, we are living in an age of hope.

It is a particularly good time to be a pediatric neurosurgeon. Major advances in technology have enabled us to do things in the OR that could not be done even a few decades ago. Antibiotics, steroids, and anti-seizure medications have made surgery safer. Microsurgical magnification and adjuncts, including diffusion tensor imaging of fiber tracts, intraoperative ultrasonography and MRI, computer-based frameless stereotactic navigation, and intraoperative neurophysiologic monitoring, have improved the efficacy of many formidable neurosurgical procedures. Advances in optics and miniaturization have allowed certain neurosurgical cases to be performed using endoscopes and miniaturized instruments with minimal invasiveness. Some brain tumors that were once considered inoperable can now be resected and even cured. For those that cannot be removed surgically, improvements in molecular neuropathology have opened a discipline of personalized medicine to improve outcomes, identifying genetic tumor alterations that can be targeted with drugs that may prove to be more effective and less toxic than conventional treatments.

But technology comes with a price—and the price is not purely monetary. If not managed appropriately, technology has the potential to drive a wedge between the doctor and patient. Technological progress is focused more on treating the disease than on healing the patient. As a result, there can be a tendency to diminish the importance of the role of the physician at the bedside—of bedside diagnosis and bedside manner—along with other humanitarian measures in medicine.

The field of medicine has changed dramatically in recent years, as anyone who has tried to make an appointment to see their own doctor for a medical problem or a routine checkup is aware. Physicians conducting clinic visits are sometimes so busy entering data into the computer's electronic health record (EHR) that they end up treating the patient as an illness rather than a person. In some instances, the physician will even bring in a scribe to enter details of the encounter into the computer in real time, further diluting the intimate relationship between doctor and patient. The doctor has become a *health-care provider*, and the patient has become a *client*. The sacred bond between doctor and patient ends up weakened.

What has happened to the laying on of the hands, one of the doctors' oldest skills for connecting with their patients? And what about the give-and-take and back-and-forth between doctor and patient that used to be so common? In some sense, they have taken a back seat to the powerful computer. And the novel video telemedicine visits, which became hugely popular in the COVID-19 pandemic, create another problem. Certainly, they are practical for many patients, particularly those who live far from the medical center. But they create an additional barrier by eliminating completely the laying on of the hands, along with other aspects of the physical examination.

The EHR is an example of the power of technology and the importance of harnessing it appropriately. For example, the EHR uses a coding system called the International Classification of Diseases (ICD) that is universally accepted by the medical community and insurance providers. But somewhere along the way, technology got out of control. So much data has been generated that it is often hard to find the key points that matter.

Medical providers are being overwhelmed with information, much of which is inconsequential.

Some of the ICD-10 codes in the system are actually absurd. Did you know, for example, that there exists a code V97.33XD for *sucked into a jet engine, subsequent encounter?* Or W55.29XA for *other contact with a cow, initial encounter*? Or V91.07XA for *burn due to water-skis on fire, subsequent encounter?* These are real codes! You can google them. Somewhere along the line, someone got a little too carried away. This is information overload at its worst.

And the lengthy patient notes in the EHR, a system that was designated for *meaningful use*, have, in many cases, become almost *meaningless*. Large portions of the medical notes are copied and pasted into rigid auto-populated templates by resident physicians from one day to the next, generating a tremendous amount of data, most of which is unreadable.

In this book, I have attempted to demonstrate the balance between science and art in patient care. I have emphasized the importance of nontechnical factors in the process of healing. Advances in medicine and surgery have been extraordinary, but they must be utilized with a measure of common sense. In my own field, surgical judgment is as important as surgical technique. Does the patient with an abnormal MRI really need an operation? Is there a way to treat the problem without surgery? If surgery is necessary, what is the safest way to carry it out? Surgical judgment is both a science and an art. In the words of Ronald Weinstein, the eminent American pathologist who founded the field of telepathology, "A fool with a tool is still a fool."

This book brings readers to the bedside of real-life patients I have cared for over the years at three different medical centers: Rainbow Babies and Children's Hospital/Case Western

Reserve University School of Medicine in Cleveland, Ohio; Boston Children's Hospital/Harvard Medical School in Boston, Massachusetts; and my current position at Johns Hopkins Children's Hospital in Baltimore, Maryland. Names have not been changed, and are used with permission. Many of the narratives are gut-wrenching.

I have also tried to illuminate the majestic complexity of the human nervous system for both the casual and the medically savvy reader. I hope to convey the wonder of unraveling the mysteries of clinical diagnosis and the pleasure of helping patients and their families navigate troubled waters that lie ahead.

I share what I have learned about the human factors—including kindness, empathy, compassion, optimism, humor, and hope—that have been critical to the process of healing for my patients. Their stories are about celebrating life and postponing death, and the mixture of human emotions associated with each profound experience. To me, these stories are far more compelling than any of the fictional tales that appear in the movies or on television. It is a great privilege to be a pediatric neurosurgeon and share the lives and dreams of so many courageous young patients. They have taught me more about the art of healing than I could ever have learned from books.

The value of human factors in healing is exemplified by the life's work of American physician Edward Livingston Trudeau. Trudeau was born in New York City in 1848. (He was the great-grandfather of the cartoonist Garry Trudeau.) When Trudeau was a teenager, he cared for his older brother James, who had contracted tuberculosis. James died after several months. Trudeau completed medical school at Columbia University in 1871 but developed tuberculosis himself two years later, shortly after returning from his honeymoon. It was a time when there was no available antimicrobial treatment for the disease.

So, Trudeau moved to the Adirondack Mountains in upstate New York for a regimen of rest, cold mountain air, and a healthy diet. Unexpectedly, he improved, enough that he was able to establish the Adirondack Cottage Sanitarium at Saranac Lake. Tuberculosis patients came in droves, including the renowned author Robert Louis Stevenson, for the uniquely compassionate care delivered by their "beloved physician." Trudeau had a huge practice where he championed the value of optimism in medicine. He spoke about it in his presidential address to the Congress of Physicians and Surgeons in Washington, DC, in May 1910.

After Trudeau's death at the age of sixty-seven in 1915, 1,200 of his grateful patients collected $7,500 and commissioned a memorial statue in his honor. The bronze on marble statue, which still stands today, was created by the Danish American sculptor Gutzon Borglum. Borglum is best remembered for carving Mount Rushmore on the granite pillars in the Black Hills of South Dakota from 1927 to 1941. The memorial statue he was hired to carve shows Trudeau in a reclining pose wrapped in a thick blanket. The base of the statue bears an inscription in French of one of Trudeau's most favorite quotes. It likely comes from the French barber surgeon of the 1500s Ambroise Paré, considered by some to be the father of modern surgery, and aptly describes the art of medicine:

> "*Guérir quelquefois, soulager souvent, consoler toujours.*"
>
> (To cure sometimes, to relieve often, to comfort always.)

CHAPTER 1

Words

"It is the province of knowledge to speak, and it is the privilege of wisdom to listen."

OLIVER WENDELL HOLMES, 1872
THE POET AT THE BREAKFAST TABLE

The vibrancy of memory is fleeting and fades with time. But some matters take on a life of their own and are unforgettable. The remarkable story of David Robinson is one that has been indelibly etched in my mind. And even though over a quarter of a century has passed since I met him, I remember things as if they had happened yesterday.

In the spring of 1997, David was a lanky, six-foot-four, straight-A high school senior with a perfect attendance record. He had excelled in math and science and played trumpet in the marching band. Life was good. He had been accepted to the college of his choice and had made plans to major in forensic chemistry. On the morning of Saturday, May 17, his spirits were riding high. He and his family had organized a visit to Ohio

University, the institution where he would begin his freshman year the following month. Because it was some distance away from home, they drove there the day before and stayed overnight in a motel.

David woke up the next morning and had an early breakfast with his parents, Michael and Paula, and his younger brother, Jeffrey. He was eager to join the college marching band and had scheduled a visit with the bandleader while his family toured the campus.

The meeting started off well. The band leader described when practices would be held and where the band would be performing during the school year. But as time went on, David began to feel ill. He remembered waking up that morning with a headache, which was unusual for him. He never really got headaches. The headache was bad enough that his dad gave him some Tylenol, though that didn't help. Things continued to worsen as the meeting went on, and David became sleepy and nauseated. When he went to say goodbye to the bandleader, he noticed that his right wrist felt limp, and he was barely able to shake the bandleader's hand. He met up with his family and felt so awful that he asked his parents to cut the rest of the visit short and drive him home. They obliged.

During the car ride home, David deteriorated further. His mother, father, and brother sat in the front seat so that he could lie down in the back. His headache increased, and he placed a cold can of soda against his forehead to ease the pain. It didn't help. He vomited profusely into a bag and became sleepier. Michael looked back at him through the rearview mirror and saw that he was pale and that his face was asymmetric. The right side of his mouth was drooping. Michael immediately decided to abort the long trip home and drive to the nearest hospital.

In the emergency room, David vomited again and was barely arousable. He had been dressed casually in jeans and a T-shirt. The ER team cut off his clothes and put a gown on him. His parents initially thought that he had a bad case of the flu. Both David's mother and brother had recently recovered from the flu. But now, things started to look more ominous. David developed a dense right hemiparesis (half-body weakness), barely able to move his right side.

Rammy Gold, the local neurosurgeon, was called in. Dr. Gold was concerned that there was a serious intracranial problem involving the left side of David's brain and ordered an emergency computed tomography (CT) scan. This showed a large hemorrhagic mass with focal areas of calcification in the left parietal lobe of the brain. The parietal lobe is one of the four major sections of the brain, situated above the temporal lobe between the frontal and occipital lobes. It has a major role in integrating sensory perception. The mass was so large that it extended over to the right cerebral hemisphere as well.

It is extremely unusual for a healthy teenager to develop a spontaneous cerebral hemorrhage. David had never really been sick before. Spontaneous cerebral hemorrhages are more common in adults and can sometimes be caused by rupture of abnormal blood vessels associated with hypertension. To search for the source of David's bleeding, Dr. Gold ordered a cerebral angiogram, an X-ray study in which contrast dye is injected through the femoral artery in the groin to visualize the blood vessels supplying the brain. One of the more common causes of spontaneous cerebral hemorrhage in a child is rupture of an underlying arteriovenous malformation (AVM), a congenital abnormal tangle of arteries and veins that can sometimes burst.

But the angiogram was negative. There was no AVM. It wasn't clear what had caused the large blood clot. Dr. Gold's presumptive diagnosis was that it was likely due to bleeding into a tumor in the dominant hemisphere of David's brain. He went to meet with the family to discuss plans.

I knew Dr. Gold well. He was a highly capable neurosurgeon. I call him by his first name, Rammy, because years earlier, he was a trainee of mine. He was also a very personable guy—bright, jovial, easygoing, larger than life. His presence would usually light up a room. But this time, things were different. The matter was serious, and Rammy was deeply apprehensive.

He knew that David would need urgent surgery, but he was concerned that the operation was too complex to be done at his hospital. At the same time, he wasn't sure that David was stable enough to be transferred to a tertiary medical center. It was a frank, difficult discussion he had with the family. The encounter was later described to me in detail by David's distraught parents, who had spent the day at their son's bedside watching him progressively worsen. They called it the worst day of their lives.

Rammy put up the CT scan on a lightbox and began describing the findings. The parietal lobe tumor was hard to miss—it stood out as an irregular, round, massive, grayish-white glob. On seeing it, David's brother, Jeffrey, promptly fainted and fell to the floor. He was placed on a stretcher and resuscitated by the ER staff. Michael and Paula were beside themselves. They had begun the day with a joyous visit to their older child's future college and, hours later, found themselves in the emergency room of a strange hospital watching him slip into a coma.

There was no warmup. Michael and Paula had no prior experience with brain surgery. David had always led a charmed life. His parents were overwhelmed with grief and were afraid he was going to die. They were in shock. They tried to block out the thought of losing their child. A nun came to visit them in the ER. "We wanted her to get lost," Michael told me. Although they were a devout Catholic family, they were terrified and had no interest in last rites. They refused to speak to the nun and waved her away abruptly.

Rammy called me on the phone and told me about the case. We arranged to transfer David to our medical center, Rainbow Babies and Children's Hospital/Case Western Reserve University in Cleveland, Ohio, immediately by helicopter with a life flight team. The family made the two-hundred-mile trip separately by car.

I went to the hospital to see David when he arrived late in the evening. He was in bad shape, and his exam was just as Rammy had described. I ordered a contrast-enhanced magnetic resonance image (MRI), a study that gave a clearer picture of the large, deep-seated hemorrhagic tumor. We admitted David to the pediatric intensive care unit (PICU) and placed him on dexamethasone, a steroid, to help reduce the swelling around the tumor and decrease the intracranial pressure. We added phenytoin, a medication to prevent seizures, and made plans for surgery the following morning.

It was late when I went to meet the family, and I was tired. It had clearly been a long day for everyone. Michael and Paula were physically and emotionally exhausted. I reviewed the scans with them and told them I thought David had sustained a hemorrhage into a large tumor deep in his brain. He needed urgent surgery. I explained in detail why and how we were going to operate. I obtained the requisite informed consent after going over the surgical risks, which were formidable. The situation was worrisome, and the discussion was honest and blunt. I could see the fear in their eyes and attempted to bring the temperature in the room down.

"I'm a neurosurgeon, but I'm also the father of two boys, though my kids are younger than yours," I told them. "I believe I have some idea about what you must be feeling. I'm sure it must be overwhelming. But in cases like this, the decision is straightforward. It's not an elective procedure like a facelift or nose job. There's really no other way to handle the problem."

"This is my son we're talking about," Michael said, "and I've only just met you. I don't know who you are. We're scared out of our wits. Can you help me get a second opinion? We don't know what to do."

It was after midnight, and David was in bad shape.

"I'm sorry, but there's no time for that," I told him. "We have to move quickly. We feel comfortable handling the problem here. If you have anyone you want me to talk to, I'd be happy to do that. I don't think David is stable enough to transfer elsewhere." We spoke a bit longer and went over plans again. Michael agreed and signed the consent.

The next morning, Sunday, May 18, 1997, we removed the tumor through a left parietal craniotomy in an eight-hour operation with David asleep under general endotracheal anesthesia. I was working with my skillful chief resident, Christopher Taylor (see Appendix: Where Are They Now?). We used computer-based image guidance to localize the deep-seated mass. This technique of frameless stereotactic navigation is derived from the pre-op MRI and takes advantage of computer technology to translate the two-dimensional anatomy of the MRI into the three-dimensional workspace of the OR. It's something like a GPS for the brain, enabling the surgical team to find the safest corridor to work through. Because the tumor was adjacent to the left motor cortex, the part of the brain that controls movement of the right side of the body, we used neurophysiological monitoring with electrodes on the brain to help ensure the integrity of David's motor pathways while he was asleep.

We performed the procedure with microsurgical instruments under magnification provided by a high-resolution microscope. The brain was swollen, and the tumor was angry, reddish-gray, and vascular. It was partially adherent to the falx cerebri, a strip of fibrous tissue that separates the two hemispheres of the brain. Ultimately, after a long slog in the OR, we were able to get a gross total removal of the tumor.

The anesthetic was reversed, and David was extubated. He woke up in the PICU with his parents by his side. He was stunned and asked them what was going on. He had no idea he had just undergone brain surgery and had only a vague recollection of the events of the prior day. His throat was irritated from the endotracheal tube.

"Here, take a look, David," Michael said, holding up a mirror in front of him. "You just had an operation on your brain. They took out a big tumor."

David looked and saw the large white turban on his head and noticed he had a crooked smile. The right side of his face was drooping.

"Oh my God. What happened? What's going on? You weren't kidding," he said, still not sure of how this had all transpired.

Michael and Paula breathed a sigh of relief. They were overjoyed that their son had survived the operation and was awake and able to talk.

A postoperative MRI confirmed that the tumor had been removed. Our neurosurgical team made rounds and visited David several times each day during his recuperation. On the first day after surgery, David was able to eat and was in good spirits, even cracking jokes with our team. His right-sided weakness was starting to improve.

I examined David on rounds and checked his cognitive functioning. His speech was normal. But when I asked him to subtract four from seven, I was met with a blank stare. I asked again twice, but he was unable to do that simple task. Then I asked him several other easy math problems and realized that he was completely unable to add or subtract. With further testing, I found that although he was able to speak, he couldn't read or write. His friends had sent him get-well cards, and while he could see the words, he had no idea what they meant.

"Doc, what's going on?" Michael asked me. "My son was a math genius, and now he can't subtract four from seven? And he can't read or write? What happened? Is he gonna get better?"

We were all surprised, and this was troubling.

"Yes, I think he will improve," I said, with some degree of confidence, even though I wasn't sure I was right. "I suspect the problem is related to post-op edema, swelling around the site of the tumor resection that we can see on the MRI. We're giving David steroids in his IV, and as the swelling goes down, I'm hoping his symptoms will improve."

It was a scary few days. Completely uncharted territory for the family. And there's nothing worse for a surgeon than to see a patient with a new neurologic deficit after surgery. It was a problem that he didn't have before and one that could possibly have been caused by a technical error, a surgical misadventure. Every surgeon carries with him or her a list of the complications they had a role in causing. It's a list that no surgeon ever forgets.

Mercifully, David's symptoms resolved. Completely. They were likely secondary to the post-operative edema (swelling), which also ultimately went away. We all breathed easier.

David's post-op symptoms and signs were a variant of a unique neurological condition called Gerstmann syndrome. It is one of the most remarkable presentations in all of neurology. The full-blown syndrome consists of four bizarre findings: agraphia (inability to write), acalculia (inability with arithmetic), finger agnosia (inability to identify fingers), and right/left disorientation. Some patients have difficulty reading as well.

Gerstmann syndrome is localized to the parietal lobe of the dominant hemisphere of the brain, the precise location of David's tumor. Specifically, Gerstmann syndrome appears to come from an insult to the lower portion of the dominant parietal lobe, the angular and supramarginal gyri in the inferior parietal lobule. The condition was described in 1924 by Josef Gerstmann, an Austrian-born neurologist working at the University of Vienna, who saw this tetrad of findings in a few of his patients. It's no small feat that he was able to describe this in an era way before conventional neuroimaging with CT and MRI.

Gerstmann was persecuted as a Jew by the Nazis and was thrown out of the University of Vienna in April 1938. He emigrated to the United States, where he spent the rest of his career, initially in Springfield, Ohio, and subsequently in New York City in private practice with an office on Central Park South.

In a tertiary medical center, our patients also serve as our teachers. We discuss neurological findings with the residents and medical students on rounds every day. A lot of medical and surgical training occurs at the bedside. Clinical correlations like this offer a powerful opportunity for teaching the complexities of neuroanatomy, which can be an exceedingly dry subject.

Thankfully, David's Gerstmann syndrome was transient and ultimately resolved as his brain swelling went away.

William Osler, the father of modern medicine, recognized the importance of bedside diagnosis and teaching over a century ago. In 1889, he left his post as chair of clinical medicine at the University of Pennsylvania and moved to Baltimore to become one of the four founding professors at my institution, the newly opened Johns Hopkins Hospital, the place where I currently work. He served as its first physician-in-chief and became a professor of medicine at the Johns Hopkins University School of Medicine, which opened in 1893. He was a legendary physician who developed the first medical residency training program in America. He was the first to bring medical students out of the lecture hall to the bedside.

Osler famously said, "He who studies medicine without books sails an uncharted sea, but he who studies medicine without patients does not go to sea at all." Those words ring true over a century later.

Meanwhile, David received inpatient physical and occupational therapy, and his hemiparesis resolved. But Michael and Paula's anxiety level remained high. To add to their anxiety, the tumor was very rare, and we couldn't tell for sure right away whether it was malignant or benign. What did the biopsy show? What type of tumor was it? What happens next? The answers were not simple and didn't come quickly. Large brain tumors that bleed have abnormal blood vessels and are often malignant—that is, cancerous.

"Is it cancer?" Michael asked me.

"We can't tell yet," I said hesitantly. "The pathologists are running special stains and working on it."

Because David's tumor was so atypical, our neuropathologists sent the specimens out to another institution for a second opinion. It took longer than a week to confirm the diagnosis. It was a tormenting week. The nail-biting wait for Michael and Paula was almost unbearable.

"Ganglioglioneurocytoma," I announced, trying not to mispronounce the tongue twister. "That's a mouthful. It's a rare mixed tumor containing neurons (nerve cells) and glia (Latin for "glue"), which are the brain's supporting cells. The tumor is benign," I said, finally able to deliver some good news. "It's not cancer."

Michael and Paula hugged each other and wept. The post-op meeting with the parents after a neurosurgical operation on their child is always intense. The level of emotion in the room is off the wall. The family must sit at the edge of their chairs and wait for potentially ominous news about their precious child. This conversation is one of the most riveting experiences a pediatric neurosurgeon can ever have. It is always deeply personal. And it always ends with tears, happy or sad. The bond that develops between the pediatric neurosurgeon and the patient and family is powerful, often lifelong.

A few days after David's surgery, his father, Michael, came to my office in the hospital and met with my secretary, Helen. Helen is a force of nature with a firecracker personality and a heart of gold. People love talking to her and find it easy to confide in her. She has an emotional IQ that's off the scale.

Michael recounted the events that brought them to the hospital and described his first encounter with me.

"It was after midnight. I was told, 'There's the doctor you need to talk to.' And here's a fellow in a blue shirt and a blazer with his hair all messed up, wearing jeans and loafers with no socks and, you know, my first thought is, I've got the Saturday night guy. The guy who gets all the calls that nobody wants, and he was home with his feet up watching TV and somebody called him and said, 'Doc, you gotta come down to the hospital. We got some poor kid being life-flighted here.'"

Michael was still overcome with emotion and still reeling over the events of the prior weekend. He's a genuinely kind soul with reddish brown hair, a powerful build, and strong hands. But he began to break down as he continued to tell Helen what it felt like the night before surgery.

"We were scared out of our minds. There isn't any way to explain it. I mean you take your child's life, and you hand it over to someone you just met, and you're totally helpless to have anything to do with what happens." Even now, it's hard to imagine how terrifying the experience must have been for Michael and Paula.

A month after surgery, David was able to attend his high school graduation, where he received a standing ovation from his classmates when he walked on stage, bald-headed, with his surgical scar in full view, to accept his diploma. Over the next several weeks, he made a complete recovery and is living a great life.

David is now in his forties, happily married with three kids of his own. He has a high-priority position in the Department of Defense at the National Geospatial Intelligence Agency with a job clearance level I'm not privileged to know. His wife, Nikole, works for the same organization. He can subtract four from seven with ease and has no difficulty with the high-powered math required in his profession. I've enjoyed a wonderful relationship with David and his parents, and we've exchanged letters and calls during the holidays over the years. His follow-up MRIs have remained clean, and we consider the surgery to be a technical success.

The pediatric neurosurgeon's role is not just to operate and remove the tumor, but to help the patient and family navigate through the process of the illness. The art of healing requires much more than the technical ability to perform surgery. It requires an understanding of who the patient is and how the patient is dealing with the stress of what is often a daunting illness. It requires the surgeon to understand the importance of empathy and compassion in helping the patient cope with a life-changing experience.

Osler, who spoke and wrote eloquently, reminded his trainees, "The good physician treats the disease; the great physician treats the patient who has the disease."

Along the same lines, technology treats the disease, but humanity heals the patient. And humanity is important in healing the entire family as well.

When doctors talk to patients and their families, there is always a delicate balance between honesty and hope. The wise physician will understand that honesty can be carried out with compassion so as not to mitigate the healing power of hope. I had been practicing neurosurgery for over a decade at the time and felt comfortable with my interpersonal skills. I was even teaching a course about Breaking Bad News for the medical students and resident trainees.

But in retrospect, I wish I could have done a better job walking Michael and Paula through what was the greatest crisis of their lives. On the night of our first meeting, it seems as if I came off tone-deaf. I didn't listen carefully enough to what Michael and Paula were going through. In the art of doctoring, the ability to listen is at least as important as choosing the right words to say. While getting consent for the surgery, I was reviewing standard operative risks and ticking off possibilities of stroke, weakness, paralysis, blindness, and more, while Michael and Paula were wondering whether they would ever see their son alive again. They were incapacitated with fear. I should have done a better job choosing my words to help comfort them through the terrible ordeal.

The influence of words in medicine has been under-recognized. Words are powerful in all social interactions and can be particularly effective in the art of healing. In 1923, the English novelist Rudyard Kipling made the point succinctly in an address to the Royal College of Surgeons in London: "Words are, of course, the most powerful drug used by mankind."

Technology has led to tremendous strides in medicine and surgery. It allowed us to find our way through the complex neural networks in David Robinson's brain and safely excise his large tumor. But technology has its limitations. If not managed correctly, technology can create a wall between the doctor and patient—and between the doctor and the patient's family.

Words can help heal. The importance of empathy in medicine is paramount. Empathy is the act of being troubled by another's trouble. It is the ability to identify and understand the emotions of others. Empathy is a difficult concept to describe, and there is no standard formula for expressing it. Trying to define empathy reminds me of the words of former Supreme Court Justice Potter Stewart describing pornography: "I know it when I see it."

On a lighter note, words must be taken in context. I have a vivid recollection of the importance of context dating back to my residency training at Bellevue. Over the years, the hospital staff had come to know me in my daily outfit of blue surgical scrubs and white OR clogs. One day, I was giving a lecture and came dressed in a suit and tie. I was in a crowded elevator, which stopped on the floor of the OR. As the door opened, one of the

OR nurses looked at me and promptly said, "Oh, Dr. Cohen, I didn't recognize you with your clothes on." Then the elevator door closed. I turned beet red and realized that there was nothing I could say to the crowd around me to clarify the situation.

Empathy is a component of caring. On October 21, 1926, Francis Weld Peabody, professor of medicine at Harvard Medical School and director of the Thorndike Memorial Laboratory, addressed the student body about the importance of empathy. His words still resonate: "The secret of the care of the patient is in caring for the patient."

No two people express empathy the same way. But when it's not there, patients and families feel its absence. Caring, comforting, compassion. These are essential but not exclusive ingredients in the art of healing. Technology facilitates the process of treatment; compassion promote the process of healing.

CHAPTER 2

Mistaken Identity

"Things are seldom what they seem;
Skim milk masquerades as cream."

Little Buttercup
from William Schwenck Gilbert and
Arthur Seymour Sullivan
H.M.S. Pinafore, May 25, 1878

On a cool sunny afternoon in September of 2015, I was in my office at Boston Children's Hospital/Harvard Medical School doing some mundane charting on the electronic health record (EHR). I was on call and was typing notes into the computer about patients I had seen on rounds earlier in the day. Charting on the EHR has always been one of my least favorite activities. In one sense, the EHR has really been a major technological breakthrough, enabling physicians to rapidly document and share digital information about their patients, improving quality, safety, and efficiency. In another sense, it has become a sterile, bulky, automated coding and billing generator.

My email inbox lit up with a message from Mark Kieran, the chief of pediatric neuro-oncology. A woman from Florida had written him requesting a second opinion about her infant daughter, who had been diagnosed with an inoperable malignant brain tumor. He thought the MRIs she had attached appeared unusual and asked if I would take a look and give her a call.

The MRIs were unusual indeed. There was a giant, contrast-enhancing solid and cystic, angry-looking tumor that occupied most of the left hemisphere of the infant's brain. It caused significant brain compression, pushing structures from the left side of the brain across the midline to the right. It was a life-threatening tumor. I remember thinking that if something that size were in my brain, I wouldn't be alive.

Adult skulls are fixed, rigid boxes that contain only the brain, the blood, and the cerebrospinal fluid. There's no room for anything else. But infants' skulls are different, consisting of multiple bones separated by cranial sutures—open growth plates. This allows the baby's head to pass through the birth canal at the time of delivery and enables the brain to grow during childhood. The cranial sutures fuse after several years to complete the rigid skull. These open cranial sutures can also act as safety valves for infants with brain tumors, allowing the head to expand and accommodate the extra mass. This is why one of the telltale signs of an infant brain tumor is macrocephaly, an enlarged head.

The baby's name was Abigail Jones, and she was only a few weeks old. I called her mother, Erika, on the phone to get the details. Erika was extremely medically savvy, as she worked as a neurology/neurosurgery nurse at the local medical center. I sat back and listened to her remarkable story.

Erika had recently given birth to Abigail, her second child, after a complicated pregnancy. Erika had been in excellent health, and the pregnancy was going along smoothly until the eighteenth week of gestation. A fetal ultrasound showed several concerning findings. A cell-free DNA blood test was performed that confirmed the diagnosis of trisomy 21, Down syndrome.

Down syndrome is the most common genetic disorder in humans and affects over five million people worldwide. Typically, healthy babies are born with forty-six chromosomes, threadlike proteins in the nuclei of our cells that carry the essential genetic information. We inherit twenty-three chromosomes from our mother and twenty-three from our father. In Down syndrome, there's an extra copy, partial or complete, of chromosome 21 in each cell of the body, increasing the total number of chromosomes in the cell's nucleus from forty-six to forty-seven. This extra chromosome can lead to a variety of distinctive physical and intellectual challenges.

The syndrome was first identified by an English physician, John Langdon Down, in 1866, and was subsequently named for him. Aside from that alarming diagnosis, Erika's fetus was otherwise strong and viable. Erika and her husband, Stephen, had made the decision to continue the pregnancy. They had no question about their decision. They were filled with love for their unborn child.

However, more tough news was to come. At thirty weeks' gestation, a repeat fetal ultrasound showed a large tumor filling the left hemisphere of Abigail's brain. That was an ominous finding, particularly because a fetal ultrasound performed four weeks earlier had shown no tumor at all. Two weeks later, a fetal MRI done with Abigail still in her mother's uterus confirmed the presence of the large tumor and delineated the abnormalities more graphically. Even worse, the MRI demonstrated that the tumor had enlarged significantly over the prior two weeks.

Erika and Stephen had a series of frank meetings with their doctors. The diagnosis of an aggressive-appearing fetal neoplasm (tumor) filling one hemisphere of the brain was extremely worrisome. Out of an abundance of compassion, the doctors advised that once the baby was born, Erika and Stephen should take her home immediately for hospice care. Their advice made sense. This was a rapidly enlarging, inoperable, malignant fetal brain tumor. The child was not expected to survive, and the staff didn't want Erika and Stephen to spend the limited time they would have with their baby in a hospital intensive care unit before she died.

Abigail was born via cesarean section at thirty-eight weeks' gestation, two weeks before term. She weighed eight pounds eleven ounces. She had diffusely low muscle tone and was taking feedings very poorly. A nasogastric feeding tube was inserted to give her nutrition. A repeat MRI on the day she was born showed that the daunting left-hemisphere brain tumor had continued to enlarge. Erika and Stephen took their newborn daughter home planning for her anticipated death.

Erika created a detailed diary and shared with me the powerful words she wrote in a blog she posted about their journey:

> "I spent the next hour choking back tears kneeling in front of my baby, asleep in the swing, just pleading that she won't leave me. So hard to read her medical reports and accept. I know what they say, I've only read them 100x, but it's still so hard to see it printed there in black and white. With "Jones, Baby Girl" listed as the patient. My heart throbs and I cannot breathe reading it. According to the most recent MRI report, the tumor measures 10 cm front to back,

> 7 cm left to right, 7.5 cm up and down. 10 cm!! For the first time, I got out a tape measure to see exactly how big that is and the answer is really stinking big. Especially next to Abigail's head. The report is so terribly bleak I can hardly stand to read it. I look at her, and I just can't understand, can't believe this report is about my Abigail. Something has got to be wrong here."

It is hard to imagine the anguish these young parents must have endured while preparing to bury their newborn child. But Erika and Stephen had worked through a lot of the issues with Abby's caregivers and had steeled themselves to be emotionally prepared. They were grateful for the brief time they would get to spend with their beautiful daughter. A photography friend gave them a gift of a heartfelt photo shoot of Abby, which they posted on the internet. It went viral. They had a series of lovely visits from friends and family, who brought them so much food that Erika didn't have to cook for several months.

At home, Abby was listless and fed poorly. She continued to require nasogastric tube feedings. Erika and Stephen hired a hospice nurse who came over a few times each week. They had a birthday party for Abby every week, not knowing how long she would survive. They made no appointments for newborn visits or vaccinations. They were devout Christians and decided Abby's middle name would be *Noelle*, derived from the Latin *natalis dies Domini*, which means "birthday of the Lord," because they felt all her future birthdays would be in heaven. They took her to the beach so she could touch the sand and ocean. They thought the next time they'd visit the beach would be to spread her ashes.

Erika posted on her blog:

> "We have been told since I was 30 weeks pregnant that our baby was going to die. We've been through all the emotions. I've envisioned her death a thousand times, watched her die a thousand ways. Lost night after a night of sleep, afraid to lay her down, to close my eyes, paranoid she's going to take her last breath without me. I've planned her funeral, what we would do with her ashes, what songs we would sing, what pictures I would display to show how perfect she was and how much she was loved.
>
> I've practiced how to tell the world we lost her, without losing it myself. I refused baby gifts, dreading I'd have to return them without a baby to use them. I've left tags on clothes, gifts still in their bags, older baby toys handed down from big sister Audrey still packed up. Abigail has no nursery, no cute room especially designed for her. In fact, I have no idea where she'll sleep when she has outgrown the bassinet.
>
> We haven't planned that far ahead. In an effort to guard my heart, I've made every attempt to prepare for Abigail's impending death. A lifetime is a lifetime, no matter how long or short it is. And we are determined to make Abigail's lifetime incredibly fulfilling and joyful. She will know how loved she is."

Slowly, things began to take a turn. As an experienced neurology/neurosurgery nurse, Erika expected the rapidly growing brain tumor to cause a swift increase in Abby's head circumference. But that never happened. In fact, Erika thought Abby's head got a little smaller. And over the next few weeks, Abby became a little more alert and interactive. After spending three weeks at home, she no longer required the nasogastric tube and began taking oral feedings, albeit slowly. A repeat MRI showed no further progression of the large tumor and suggested that it might have gotten a little smaller.

"Something didn't feel right," Erika told me.

The home hospice nurse agreed and suggested that Erika get a second opinion. The news media had picked up the photo shoot that they had posted. Erika got a message from a stranger on Facebook. The stranger was a woman whose baby was diagnosed with an inoperable fetal brain tumor that turned out to be a teratoma, a tumor that was successfully removed. The woman directed Erika to our hospital.

"How's Abby getting along today?" I asked Erika over the phone.

"She's sitting here right next to me," she said. "She's the chillest baby ever. I'm confused. She doesn't seem to be getting any worse. She's started taking feedings, and she's gaining weight. She's resting comfortably and seems fairly alert. She watches your face and tracks with her eyes."

I was surprised as well. Things didn't make sense. One of the earliest lessons I learned in my career as a pediatric neurosurgeon was to *always listen to mom*. A mother knows her child better than anyone in the world. She can pick up subtle changes that might be overlooked by seasoned medical providers, who only see the child for short periods at a time. On several occasions, I have witnessed a mother's intuition outsmart our CT scans or MRIs in determining whether her child had a neurosurgical problem, for example, malfunction of a ventriculoperitoneal shunt—a device we insert to treat hydrocephalus, an accumulation of water on the brain. I've been burned in the past by not paying enough attention to a mother's instincts and vowed never to let that happen again.

Maybe mom was right. Maybe Abby's case was different. She didn't appear to be following the course I had learned about in my medical training. I suggested that they come up for an in-person visit. I didn't want to create false hope, though, and cautioned Erika that most large fetal brain tumors have a very poor prognosis with an overall survival rate of only about 15 percent. Most neonates die shortly after birth, and some don't even make it to term. But we wanted to leave no stone unturned. Erika and Stephen were aware of the gravity of the situation. They were prepared for the worst. They decided to fly up for a visit.

Ten days later, Erika, Stephen, and Abby were in my office. Abby was pink and alert, an adorable newborn baby girl. I put up the MRI and showed Erika and Stephen the anatomy and geometry of the large intrinsic neoplasm that filled the left hemisphere of her brain.

"The baby doesn't seem to fit the scan we're looking at," I said, wondering if part of the clinical improvement might have been related to resorption of some intratumoral hemorrhage. "I think we should take a look in the OR. The odds are still steep, and the prognosis is still guarded. Most of these fetal brain tumors are bad actors. But something doesn't compute here. I think there's enough question about the diagnosis that we shouldn't give Abigail a death sentence."

I was reminded of something I learned at the beginning of my career from Paul Rosman, one of the finest pediatric neurologists I had ever worked with: "We treat the patient, not the X-rays."

I suggested we operate and biopsy the tumor. If it was clearly cancer and appeared unresectable, we could always stop the surgery and close up. Otherwise, we would keep going and try to remove it. Erika and Stephen liked the plan and agreed immediately. I took them on a tour of the hospital and introduced them to our team.

"Hope had been taken off the table," Erika wrote later. "Now it was back on."

Two days later, on October 8, 2015, when Abby was two months old, I was in the OR staring with disbelief at her extraordinarily unusual brain tumor. I was working with my accomplished pediatric neurosurgery fellow, Jesse Winer. We had fashioned a left frontoparietal craniotomy, elevating a piece of the skull and opening the dura mater, the fibrous lining of the brain. The brain was under pressure and was pushing out of the skull. Our eyes were fixated on a large heterogeneous mass that filled the operative bed. The tumor had multiple compartments and was brightly colored—orange, yellow, tan, green, and brown. In between the tumor septations were large cysts filled with straw-colored fluid. In several areas, the tumor was adherent to the meninges that covered the brain. The tumor was covered by a leash of abnormal blood vessels.

It certainly didn't look like cancer. We suspected that the multiple colors we saw were because the tumor had hemorrhaged, and some of what we were looking at, in addition to the tumor, was resorbing blood products. We drained the cyst cavities to reduce the intracranial pressure. We sent several biopsies of the tumor for frozen section, which was done on the spot by the neuropathologists to give us immediate feedback about the nature of the tumor.

The frozen section returned consistent with a low-grade glioneuronal tumor. The neuropathologist couldn't provide a more detailed analysis at that point. That was enough for us, though. This was not a malignant tumor. It was not cancer. So, we dug in and spent the next several hours removing it under the guidance of the operating microscope. It was a struggle, but luckily, we were able to get the entire tumor out and close up. The operation took seven and a half hours. Jesse and I were pretty tired.

Meanwhile, back in the waiting room, the anticipation was painful, and the anxiety level was high. Erika had been unable to sleep the night before. Stephen had a panic attack in the waiting room, became lightheaded and pale, and had to lie down. Erika persuaded him to go back to the hotel and cool off. She was too upset about what was going on with Abby and felt she didn't have the bandwidth to look after Stephen as well. Later in the day, the OR called into the waiting room to let Erika know that I would be coming to see them. She called Stephen on the phone, who raced back.

Meeting with the parents of a child who has just undergone surgery to remove a brain tumor is invariably one of the most intense experiences I have ever had.

"It's benign," I said, exhaling deeply. "We were able to get it all out."

Words of joy. Tears flowed from Erika and Stephen.

"What did the tumor look like?" Stephen asked me.

"It was kind of cool, like a giant oyster," I said. For some bizarre reason, neurosurgeons often describe brain tumors by comparing them to food. We all had a laugh of relief.

Years later, Erika would tell me that she and Stephen had spent months preparing for Abby to die. She told me that they were expecting bad news when I came back to talk to them so soon after starting the surgery. They thought it meant that the biopsy showed cancer and that we had to abort the procedure.

That was odd, I thought, since I was in the OR with Abby for seven and a half hours! What did they think I was doing all that time? Actually, a biopsy can be performed fairly quickly. Erika said they thought a tumor resection would have taken twice as long. In fact, sometimes it really does take twice as long. Sometimes, the OR staff teases us that they monitor our neurosurgery cases by the calendar, not the clock. No two cases are the same.

That conversation was the first time that Erika and Stephen began to prepare for their daughter to live. Things started to change rapidly. Abby was irritable after surgery and stayed in the pediatric intensive care unit for thirty-six hours. Then she turned the corner and became more alert and interactive. She never even developed significant scalp swelling. She began feeding more than she had ever done. Erika recalled, "She was eating like a horse." Part of that was likely related to the perioperative steroids she was on, and part was because the pressure on her brain had been relieved. A postoperative MRI confirmed complete removal of the tumor.

Abby was discharged from the hospital after four days. The family stayed in town for a week. They took Abby for walks around the city and for a picnic in the park. They played with her. They told me they felt as if Abby had been reborn. When they flew home, there was a crowd waiting to greet them at the airport, holding a sign: *Abigail Jones Is Going to Live!*

It took three weeks for the final pathology to come back. The diagnosis was desmoplastic infantile ganglioglioma (DIG). That is a rare benign tumor, categorized by the World Health Organization (WHO) as grade 1, the lowest and best possible score. DIG is a relatively newly described neoplasm, first reported by Scott Vandenberg and colleagues in 1987. When I was in training, the term didn't exist. The tumors existed, sure enough, but were classified as subsets of other, more common tumors, until careful clinicopathological analysis showed unique, striking features to warrant creating a new name in the WHO lexicon.

As in Abby's case, DIG tumors tend to be large, firm, cystic and solid, and involve more than one lobe of the brain, usually the frontal and parietal lobes. DIGs are usually seen in young infants, often under the age of four months. The term desmoplastic comes from desmos (Greek for "knot") and plasis (Greek for "formation") and describes the fibrous reaction of the tumor with its strong adherence to the leptomeninges (linings of the brain).

DIGs are exceedingly rare, with an incidence of less than 1 percent of all tumors of the central nervous system. These large tumors can mimic more aggressive malignancies, as was the case with Abby. I wrote an article about DIGs in the *Journal of Neurosurgery*, calling the tumor the "great neurosurgical masquerader," mistaken for other disorders. I have seen DIGs mimicking stroke, infection, and malignant tumors. It is important to consider DIG in the differential diagnosis of large, atypical brain masses in infants, as the impact on prognosis can be profound.

Abby went home with her parents and continued to thrive. She clearly has special needs. She began life with the double hits of Down syndrome and a giant brain tumor, both of which were diagnosed before she was even born. Years later she's hypothyroid and takes replacement for that. But she's not on any other medications. She has right-sided weakness related to the location of her large brain tumor. But she can cruise along furniture and walk while holding someone's hand.

Abby is eating well and relishes ice cream and finger food, particularly sweet potatoes. She loves being around family and friends. She loves to give hugs. She enjoys dancing and particularly likes the soundtracks to Disney favorites like *Moana* and *Encanto*. She's chatty and likes to sing. She lights up a room.

One hundred fifty people came to celebrate her first birthday, an event that Erika and Stephen were told would never happen.

Here again is the need to find a balance between honesty and hope. That balance is nuanced, and there is no one-size-fits-all. Hope is an essential ingredient in the bond that develops between the doctor and the family. But hope has to be tempered with honesty, as false hope, or sugarcoating, must be avoided. Mark Twain famously said, "I have too much respect for the truth to drag it out on every trifling occasion." Compassionate but honest optimism is the aspirational goal.

Abby is now eleven years old, in public school with special education classes. I keep up with the Joneses and remain in awe of their strength and stamina. I recently asked Erika to reflect on her family's experience since they got the second opinion so many years ago. I did this with some degree of apprehension, not wishing for her to have to relive the emotional trauma of eleven years earlier.

"You're asking me if I would do it again?" she asked. "Without a doubt. No question. Abby writes her own story. She has taught us to look at life differently. In a world where sorrow steals hope and joy, we know we have received a precious, irreplaceable gift. Every moment is a gift to be treasured. She may have significant special needs. Stephen and I have talked about what her quality of life might look like and if it would be worth it to put her through all of it to be severely disabled. But who are we to say what quality of life someone has? She has the ability to touch people's hearts. So, we'll take it one day at a time. She hasn't given up, and we will not give up on her."

CHAPTER 3

Grit

"Courage is grace under pressure."

Ernest Hemingway

It was late in the afternoon on Saturday, March 8, 2003, and Emma Anderson was winding down from an active day with friends at the annual Girl Scout Overnight Outing in Sandusky, Ohio. She was nine years old and in the third grade. Her mother, Julie, one of the troop leaders, was there helping oversee the event. The crowd was large, with over sixty kids immersed in a series of arts and crafts, sports activities, and games.

At about 7 p.m., Emma was relaxing with her pals in the indoor swimming pool. She was chest-deep in the water, walking across the pool, when she felt a sudden jolt of dizziness along with heaviness in both of her legs. She remembers falling underwater without being able to move her limbs or lift her head. Then she passed out.

A lifeguard was on duty but was looking elsewhere and didn't see her go down. By chance, Julie had her camera out and was taking pictures of Emma at the time. She saw Emma fall backward into the water and go under. Emma was struggling and didn't resurface. Julie screamed but could not get the lifeguard's attention. She immediately dropped her camera and jumped into the pool with her clothes on. She pulled Emma out of the water and laid her on the ground beside the pool. It was a maneuver that saved Emma's life.

Emma awakened with a crowd around her and a blood pressure cuff on her arm. She was dizzy and felt out of it, confused, and scared. She had no headache. She had never been sick before. She lay there by the pool for some time and began to feel a little better. People got her up and sat her on a bench. They were relieved she was improving and felt she had experienced an accidental near drowning.

Gradually, Emma felt well enough to join the girls for a late dinner of pizza and soda. But when she got up to go to the bathroom, she was dazed, and her legs were wobbly. She took a few steps and fell to the ground. Two Girl Scout leaders who were nearby picked her up and sat her down on a chair. Julie ran over, saw a glazed look in Emma's eyes, and panicked. She lifted Emma up, carried her to the car, and sped off to the local hospital. Emma's dad, Erik, met them in the emergency room.

Emma was on a stretcher, fluctuating in and out of consciousness. It was after midnight. The doctors examined Emma in the ER and performed a CT scan of her head. Emma remembers overhearing one of the doctors tell her parents that there was a large abnormality in the center of her brain and that things looked bad, and he wasn't sure she was going to make it. He told them that they were in a small hospital that was not equipped to deal with a problem this serious. He shook their hands, wished them luck, and shipped Emma off to our hospital in an ambulance. Julie and Erik were horrified.

They arrived at our ER at Rainbow Babies and Children's Hospital in the early hours of the morning, with Emma lethargic and unable to communicate. We got more information from her parents and learned that Emma had been complaining of unsteadiness and difficulty walking for several months, suggesting that the process had been going on for some time. On physical exam, she was stuporous.

Ophthalmologic testing showed bilateral papilledema—elevation of her optic discs because of increased intracranial pressure. Her left pupil was enlarged, a worrisome sign suggestive of an oculomotor nerve palsy with incipient transtentorial brain herniation. The oculomotor nerve (cranial nerve 3) arises from the brainstem, innervates muscles that move the eye, and causes pupillary constriction. Pupillary dilatation (mydriasis) in this setting can be caused by a mass (e.g., tumor) that compresses the brainstem and third cranial nerve, which can signify a life-threatening condition.

The CT scan from the outside hospital was markedly abnormal. There was a large bilateral thalamic tumor in the center of Emma's brain. The thalamus (Latin for "inner chamber, bedroom") is a paired ovoid gray matter structure located deep in the brain just on top of the brainstem. It acts as a relay station that filters sensory signals between the body and the brain. The two thalami sit on either side of the cerebral ventricles—the fluid spaces that produce, store, and transport the clear cerebrospinal fluid (CSF) that bathes, protects, and nourishes the brain. In Emma's case, the tumor was bithalamic, meaning that it arose from the brain substance and had already spread to involve both sides of the brain. It compressed the midline third ventricle, preventing egress of CSF, thereby causing a backup of ventricular CSF, or hydrocephalus.

The immediate problem for Emma was increased intracranial pressure. Her tumor was a large space-occupying mass that caused increased pressure on her brain because there was no room for it inside her skull. Added to that was the hydrocephalus, the fluid backup. With all that pressure in her head, it was somewhat surprising that she had experienced no headache.

We surmised that the near-drowning event may have been a seizure and placed Emma on an anti-seizure medication. Something needed to be done quickly to treat the increased intracranial pressure. We went to the OR emergently to insert an external ventricular drain, making a small hole in her skull and passing a soft silicone catheter into her enlarged ventricles. This brought down her elevated intracranial pressure by diverting the excess CSF that had built up into a sterile bag. We also gave her intravenous dexamethasone, a steroid, to reduce the brain swelling around her tumor.

These measures worked, and over the next day, Emma awakened and returned to her normal baseline. This bought us some time to continue the workup, which consisted of a brain MRI without and with intravenous gadolinium, a paramagnetic contrast agent that can help define certain brain tumors. The MRI delineated the three-dimensional geometry of Emma's tumor and confirmed the diagnosis of significant hydrocephalus by showing transependymal CSF—that is, fluid that passed through the ependymal wall lining the ventricles into the brain substance, indicative of increased pressure.

We suspected the tumor was an infiltrating glioma, a tumor arising from the glia (Greek for "glue"), the supporting cells of the brain. The surgical challenge was that the tumor was deep, bilateral, arising from the brain substance itself with no capsule separating it from normal brain, and infiltrative with multiple finger-like projections into the normal brain. This meant that we would need to operate to reduce the tumor burden, but it wouldn't be safe to attempt a total resection of the tumor for fear of causing irreparable harm to adjacent essential structures of her brain.

We devised a plan to perform an interhemispheric transcallosal craniotomy. The goals of surgery were threefold: to establish a tissue diagnosis, to reduce the tumor burden by taking out as much tumor as was safely possible, and to treat the hydrocephalus, the buildup of fluid in the ventricles that was currently being diverted into an external bag by a drainage tube. Assisting me in the OR was Jeremy Amps, a very capable junior resident.

So, with Emma asleep under general anesthesia in the OR, we made an incision across the top of her scalp and fashioned a craniotomy, removing a trap-door portion of the right side of her skull. The medial portion of the craniotomy was along the midline, directly over the superior sagittal sinus, the large vein that drains blood from the brain back to the heart through the internal jugular veins. Then we opened the dura mater (Latin for "tough mother"), the fibrous lining of the brain. We made the dural opening in a U-shape just adjacent to the midline and flapped it medially, taking care not to injure the superior sagittal sinus. This gave us the ability to go down to the depths of the brain between the two cerebral hemispheres without going through the brain.

Working under magnification provided by the operating microscope, we gently teased the two hemispheres apart until we saw the glistening corpus callosum (Latin for "white body"), the band of white matter fibers that connects the two sides of the brain. Creating a two-centimeter opening in the corpus callosum, we entered the cerebral ventricles, where we were able to see the tumor and resect a good portion of it. Because we were working in a small space, we removed it from the inside out, sort of like coring out an apple.

The interhemispheric transcallosal craniotomy is a workhorse procedure that provides the neurosurgeon access to deep midline structures without violating the cerebral cortex or any substantial amount of brain tissue. The approach was devised by Walter Dandy, one of the great neurosurgical pioneers, working at Johns Hopkins in the early 1900s. It was popularized by William Shucart and Bennett Stein in an article they published in the journal *Neurosurgery* in 1978. I learned the technique from Shucart, an extraordinary neurosurgeon and mentor of mine early in my career when I worked at the Floating Hospital for Infants and Children/Tufts New England Medical Center in Boston, Massachusetts. The magnified image of this interhemispheric corridor seen through a high-powered microscope gives the operator a mind-blowing view of the neurovascular structures hidden in the depths of the brain.

After resecting the tumor, we worked deeper in the ventricles, creating a third ventriculostomy, an opening at the floor of the third ventricle to short-circuit the CSF into the normal downstream pathways of the brain, bypassing the obstruction caused by the thalamic tumor. This allowed us to eventually remove the external ventricular drain, the "safety valve" we had placed to bring down the intracranial pressure when Emma was admitted.

Emma came through the surgery nicely and woke up talking and in pretty good spirits, given all that had transpired. Her parents were relieved. Julie had been sobbing every day since the incident in the swimming pool. Emma had demonstrated phenomenal strength throughout the ordeal and tried to give some of that strength to her mother.

"Mom, enough already. You have got to stop crying. I'm doing okay. This is a big deal for me. I need your help to get through it."

Those words helped Julie turn things around and begin focusing on Emma's recovery. She finally had a glimmer of hope. Although little Emma was only nine years old at the time, her spirit was indomitable. Here was the child helping guide her parents through what appeared to be an insurmountable problem.

Our children are born in innocence. As parents, we consider it our job to protect them at all costs. Yet in times of crisis, the roles are sometimes reversed. The resilience of the child can help the rest of the family navigate through the ordeal. I have seen this phenomenon on other occasions, and it is a heartwarming sight.

Emma's pathology report came back after a few days. It was an infiltrating fibrillary (stringy) astrocytoma, WHO grade 2. That's a low-grade malignancy, a form of cancer. Emma would need long-term chemotherapy to prevent the growth of the residual tumor. The chemotherapy would be administered by Chad Jacobson, John Letterio, and Duncan Stearns, her pediatric oncologists, and Deborah Gold, her pediatric neurologist. Emma was lucky to have them. Each was a national expert in the treatment of pediatric brain cancer. They would oversee her adjuvant treatment—the therapy that is initiated after surgical resection of the tumor. But each also had a special rapport with patients and families and knew how to deliver kid-friendly care, so much so that although Emma hated the toxicities of her treatments, she actually enjoyed coming to the hospital for her weekly chemotherapy.

Chemotherapy is a type of cancer treatment that uses drugs to kill or control the growth of tumor cells. Emma's chemotherapy consisted of vincristine and carboplatin. Vincristine is a vinca alkaloid derived from the Madagascar rosy periwinkle plant. It was first isolated in 1961 and was approved by the FDA in 1963. It has an anticancer effect by interfering with microtubule polymerization in the cell cycle, thereby blocking cell growth. Carboplatin is a platinum-containing alkylating agent. Its antineoplastic mechanism of action is to bind to DNA and kill cancer cells when they are in the resting state of the cell cycle. Carboplatin has been in clinical use since 1989, when it was approved by the FDA. The two drugs have different mechanisms of action and giving them together hits the tumor with a kind of one-two punch.

The challenge with chemotherapy is that these drugs all have associated side effects, some severe. Side effects include loss of appetite, fatigue, nausea, vomiting, anemia, bleeding, immunosuppression, alopecia (hair loss), and a host of others. But Emma was stalwart and slogged through the demanding treatments with exceptional strength. She remembers how difficult it was to be a young girl with no hair on her head. She wore wigs and hated them. She was often bullied by kids who didn't know any better. They had never met a classmate undergoing chemotherapy. One day, when there was a substitute teacher, a group of rowdy kids pulled off Emma's wig in gym class and sat around laughing at her. The school reacted by temporarily suspending the offenders and requiring them to write letters of apology to Emma. Emma was underwhelmed by the gesture. Julie suggested a better response would have been to have them visit the children's hospital for a tour of the pediatric cancer ward.

The number of kids who teased and mistreated Emma was small. Most of her classmates were kind and understanding. Curiously, not all her teachers were so empathetic. Emma had always been a straight A student. But several teachers gave her poor grades on her report card because of frequent absences. Her choir teacher said she did it because she "had to hold all students to the same standard." Some other teachers agreed.

Really? The same standard? That's like kicking someone while they're down. How many other kids in the class were going to the hospital for weekly chemotherapy? How many were dealing with the excruciating toxicities of chemotherapy? Julie was a tireless advocate for her daughter and made several complaints to the school principal, who, fortunately, was always sympathetic.

Emma's post-op course was not easy. She developed seizures that had to be controlled by anticonvulsant medication. Her blood counts fell, and she was admitted to the hospital for blood transfusions. She had recurrent mouth sores. Her implanted intravenous mediport clotted, and she needed treatment with Lovenox, a blood thinner, along with removal and replacement of the line. She was prone to infection after each chemotherapy administration when her white blood cell count fell very low.

Once she developed a severe viral encephalitis, an inflammation of the brain due to a viral infection. She struggled for months with headache, fever, dysarthria (slurred speech), and weakness on the left side of her body before she eventually recovered. She developed a peripheral neuropathy from her vincristine, which manifested as paresthesias, a prickly pins-and-needles sensation on her arms and legs.

"It was nasty," she said. "It felt like my skin was on fire all the time."

Emma completed a year of chemotherapy and was relieved once it stopped. She felt better. We followed her in the clinic with surveillance MRIs that remained stable. But after a year, the tumor started to grow. Even though she felt okay, she needed another year of chemotherapy. That year was just as painful as the first. Finally, after this bout, things got better, and Emma went into remission. No more painful treatments. No more transfusions. No more infections. She went back to being the normal kid she was before her tumor diagnosis.

It may be a stretch to say that Emma was really ever *normal*. She was always a remarkable child. She credits her sense of humor for helping her get through the illness. And that same sense of humor helped bring her family through the ordeal as well. The healing power of humor should not be underestimated.

Each winter in Cleveland, when the skies were gray and the weather was cold, I used to get a group of my patients together for an annual karaoke festival to celebrate the birthday of the King of Rock and Roll, Elvis Presley. We called January 8th Elvis Day. We did it to have some fun with these young kids who were hospitalized with very serious medical disorders. Many of them didn't even know who Elvis was. I would dress up in a sky-blue sateen rhinestone suit, along with sunglasses and gold platform shoes, and get the kids together in the atrium of the Children's Hospital to sing, dance, and put on a show for the patients, their families, and the hospital staff. What we lacked in talent, we made up for in enthusiasm.

One year, the Emmy-winning TV morning news show *Good Morning America* called and said they'd heard about us and wanted to come over to film the event. I told them not to bother—we had been doing this for several years and weren't very good, so the kids and I were about to hang up the microphone and retire.

"We'll be there in two weeks," the *GMA* rep said. "So, start practicing."

And so, we practiced. And they came. It was a surreal experience. There were a few hundred people in the audience, and I was uncomfortable for several reasons, not the least of which was that I could not carry a tune. But that was not the case for Emma. Even though she had never even heard of Elvis and had never been on a stage, she showed up in a black leather jacket and sunglasses and took control. She grabbed the microphone and stood out on the stage in front of everyone. She danced and belted out one song after another, imploring all the other kids and me to follow along.

It was unforgettable seeing these brave kids who were battling some of the most terrifying illnesses imaginable come together to kick back and celebrate life. Our performance subsequently aired on a *GMA* segment anchored by Diane Sawyer called "Doctor Elvis." I was relieved that the first-rate videographers at ABC were able to edit out most, though not all, of the many notes we missed. It was a blast.

For Emma, that was just the beginning. While she was undergoing cancer chemotherapy, she overheard me talking to a group of residents and medical students about a song I had written. At the time, I was teaching a course in neuroanatomy in the medical school. While the human nervous system is striking in its beauty and complexity, neuroanatomy can be one of the driest courses imaginable. A lot of it involves rote memorization, and a lot of that memorization happens in the wee hours of the night.

I remember when I was a medical student, how painful it was to sit through some of these basic science lectures. An exceptionally painful memory is of an hour-long discourse in which the professor shared with us every minute detail he had ever learned about the microscopic anatomy of the thalamus. As far as I was concerned, he might as well have been speaking Latin or Greek. Actually, for much of the talk, he was speaking in Latin and Greek. It's hard to make that material come alive in a lecture, and as a student, one's mind tends to wander. I was drifting off.

The medical researcher RK Rathbun said perceptively: "A lecture is a process by which the notes of the professor become the notes of the students without passing through the minds of either."

My classmate Dave Davis and I found a way to pass the time when the lecture material in medical school got really monotonous. We would sit next to each other in the back of the classroom and do the *New York Times* Crossword Puzzle, passing the paper back and forth to each other surreptitiously until we got it completed. But living on the edge like that came with a price.

There was one particularly dull pharmacology lecture late in the morning on a Thursday. I was sitting in the back row on the aisle, and Dave was sitting directly in front of me. I was doing the puzzle and only got about halfway through it. The *Times* Crossword gets progressively more difficult as the week goes on, and this Thursday's puzzle was a real bear. So, I finished what I could and slipped the puzzle onto Dave's desk in front of me. Little did I realize that Dave had zoned out and was completely asleep. Unfortunately, the professor did notice that something was awry and interrupted his lecture to walk up the aisle and address the problem.

"Mister Davis, if you find the need to do the crossword puzzle, perhaps it would be more appropriate if you did it on your own time rather than in my class!"

The professor didn't even realize that poor Dave was fast asleep and had no idea the partially finished puzzle was on his desk, thanks to me. I will never forget that episode.

I vowed that if I were ever going to teach medical students, I would make a strong effort to connect with my audience. I remember the clever words of the British American poet W. H. Auden, "A professor is one who talks in someone else's sleep."

So, years later, when the tables turned and I morphed from student to educator, I explored alternative methods of teaching. Instead of articulating in class everything I had learned about the microanatomy of the thalamus, I attempted to make the neuroanatomy come alive for the students, hoping that it would inspire them to go back and read about the details on their own. One way I did this was by composing a song entitled "Extreme Neuroanatomy" to the lively tune of Gilbert and Sullivan's "I Am the Very Model of a Modern Major General." This, of course, came from their acclaimed comic opera of 1879, *The Pirates of Penzance*.

"Extreme Neuroanatomy" was my humble modification of their masterpiece, updated for students of the neurosciences. It contains all the terms I deemed necessary for my trainees to know in order to become a brain surgeon. Here's a sample:

The pterion and inion and euryon and nasion

Asterion opisthion obelion and basion

And bregma lambda clivus vomer foramen ovale

Hypophysis paraphysis and corpus pineale

The basal vein of Rosenthal olfactory tuberculum

The torcular Herophili parietal operculum

And atrium ventriculi lemniscus lateralis

Forceps major basis pontis trigone nucleus basalis…

Although friends have accused me of being tone-deaf, I would sing the song for the medical school class, with background music provided on the keyboard by one of my exceptionally talented neurosurgery residents at the time, Jonathan Miller. We provided the students with a handout that defined all the terms and told them that if anyone could sing the song from memory, that individual wouldn't have to take the exam. It was a long, convoluted song, and, not unexpectedly, no one was ever able to sing it.

With one exception. That was my fearless young prodigy patient, Emma Anderson. She learned the entire song and sang it with passion to anyone who would listen. She drove her parents crazy by singing it to them multiple times a day, every day. She even boldly belted out a version to thunderous applause at one of the yearly Elvis Day celebrations at the hospital.

My point is to emphasize the role that humor can play in the healing process. As the French Enlightenment philosopher Voltaire noted, "The art of medicine consists in amusing the patient while nature cures the disease."

Humor helps with healing. Humor can reduce stress, improve pain, aid in overcoming fear, and help to provide hope. If used appropriately, humor can build trust and strengthen the bond between the doctor and the patient, especially if the patient is a child. Humor is *vitamin H*. And this is nothing new. Even the Old Testament notes, "A merry heart doeth good like a medicine" (Proverbs 17:22 KJV).

That's not to say the physician should attempt to do stand-up comedy at the bedside of a gravely ill patient in the intensive care unit. But humor has a role in medicine. And humor is especially important when dealing with kids, as it can help to make the doctor more human and strengthen the connection between doctor and child. Let your guard down. Make yourself more vulnerable. The rewards are powerful. There is no question that for Emma, her sense of humor—along with her unbreakable spirit—helped her get through a significant number of grueling adjuvant chemotherapy sessions.

I've kept up with Emma, and we have spoken to each other and written each other often. Seven years after her surgery, Julie decided to throw her a surprise Sweet Sixteen birthday party. She set it up for 6 p.m. on a weeknight at a local restaurant in her hometown, about an hour's drive from my hospital. I got an invitation from Julie and was looking forward to the event—I had not seen Emma for several years. Julie gave me strict instructions to keep everything on the down low because the party was a surprise. It was going to be a big event, with over forty people invited. Emma's sister, Erika, suggested that she dress up for the evening, which took Emma by surprise because the restaurant was a pretty low-key place. But she was game and went along with the plan. So, they dressed up and went over to have dinner.

As luck would have it, I had a late case in the OR that day and had forgotten to get directions to the restaurant. So, while I was scrubbed in for surgery, I had the OR staff call my medical assistant, Helen, and she dutifully left instructions for me on my desk. The festivities would be held at Mister Smith's Coffee House at 140 Columbus Street.

I finished the OR case, grabbed the directions, and raced off to the party. I was really moving along on the highway, but when

I got to town, I found myself driving down an unlit dirt road in the middle of nowhere with no buildings in sight. I thought to myself, This seems to be an unusual place for a restaurant. But it must have some very good food for people to come here to eat. After driving around for a bit longer, I came to the sad realization that there was no restaurant to be found. I called Julie in a panic. She told me that Helen had mistakenly sent me to Columbus *Street* but the restaurant was actually on *Columbus Avenue.* She gave me directions over the phone and stayed on with me till I got there.

I was already an hour late, and the party had begun, but Julie wanted my arrival to be a surprise, so she spoke to me from outside the restaurant. She still reminds me about that, because it was February and the night air was cold, and she wasn't wearing a coat. When I finally got there, Emma saw me from across the room, shouted "Big Al!" at the top of her lungs, and raced over to give me a big hug. Moments like that are unforgettable. It's part of the unique joy of being a pediatric neurosurgeon. The party was a huge success, and Emma had a blast. I had some words with Helen the next day, who told me she was happy to be my professional assistant, but that from then on, I would have to be responsible for my social calendar myself.

Emma has been in remission for over two decades. She has moved on with her life. She always had a passion for art and earned two trips to Disney World when her paintings won first prize in the Littlest Heroes competition. She earned a BA and a master's degree in art, and now, at age thirty-two, twenty-three years after her surgery, she teaches art to young students and holds several exhibitions of her own work each year. To make ends meet, she also works part-time as a barista at Starbucks and serves as a substitute teacher for several public elementary schools in the inner city.

Emma has always been passionate about art and has used it as a means of expressing her emotions. As a teacher, she has tried to impart that passion to her young students. But what I found most intriguing was to hear her describe her experience as a substitute teacher. It was not an easy job. And listening to her speak about it was the only time I ever heard her express fear.

Working as a substitute teacher several times a week, she has taught classes ranging from kindergarten through sixth grade. Kids can be disruptive and often take advantage of a substitute teacher by acting out in ways they would not ordinarily. Emma frequently had to deal with bullies and break up fights. One day, she remembers having to break up three fights before 9 a.m. Emma was also concerned about being around large groups of kids in case she might still be immunocompromised from her treatments.

But the main concern Emma had about teaching was what we read about all too often in the newspapers—violence, particularly the epidemic of gun violence. According to the Centers for Disease Control and Prevention, gun violence is now the number-one cause of death for American children. That is a remarkable statement. Throughout the history of our country, disease has been the number-one cause of childhood death. Decades ago, when I was growing up, the number-one cause was motor vehicle accidents. Since 2020, the number-one killer of children has been firearms, responsible for more childhood deaths than cancer, congenital anomalies, drug overdoses, poisoning, drowning, suffocation, and motor vehicle collisions.

Emma Anderson, who stared down cancer without blinking, was afraid to teach elementary school classes for fear of gun violence. She hated the virtual and in-person training sessions on gun violence she had to attend. She hated the drills with her young students with the lights off, showing them how to lock the doors and hide in the coat room without making a sound. The world has changed, and it's hard to imagine the toll this takes on our nation's young children and their teachers. Emma found it easier to go through chemotherapy.

More than two decades after her surgery, Emma has become a brain cancer survivor and is now a healthy young adult and a fierce advocate for brain cancer awareness. She is active in fund-raisers and organizes and participates in online forums to offer comfort, support, and hope for young patients who are going through what she experienced as a young child. I met up with Emma recently and asked her how the brain tumor had shaped her life. Her answer caught me by surprise.

"If I could live my life again, I would do it with cancer," she said.

"Are you crazy?" I asked, wondering if she had lost some of her marbles in the experience.

"Not at all," she replied firmly, without missing a beat. "Life sometimes throws you a curve ball. I think there must have been a reason I got cancer. From the time I got my diagnosis, I was no longer the same person I was before. Cancer has made me stronger. It made me a fighter. Cancer made me who I am today. I wouldn't change a thing."

Emma's words left me dumbstruck. She faced her destiny with incredible fortitude and tenacity. Throughout all of her treatments, she went out of her way to protect her friends and her family. She never wanted anyone to feel sorry for her. She never wanted to be a burden. Having emerged from such a difficult childhood, she has become an inspirational young woman.

Recently, a local news group in Cleveland did a feature story about Emma and asked me to come back for it. I hadn't seen her in years, and we sat together and reminisced about the old days. She smiled broadly and turned to me. "Big Al, now that we've got the band back together, why don't we do a rendition of 'Extreme Neuroanatomy'? For old time's sake."

By "got the band back together," I guess she meant the two of us. I hesitated, knowing full well that she would show me up and I'd end up embarrassed again. But she was relentless and would not take no for an answer. So, we sang together with an a cappella version of the song I had written twenty years ago. I was able to make it through three stanzas before I stumbled, forgot the words, and was unable to continue. Emma didn't flinch, completing the song alone perfectly.

"I'm sorry, Emma," I said, trying to explain away my humiliation about forgetting the words to my own song. "I've had a lot on my mind lately."

"No excuses, Big Al," she said firmly. "Come on, man. No excuses."

CHAPTER 4

Lasting Impact

"Tears come from the heart and not from the brain."

Leonardo da Vinci

The year 1999 had been a busy one for Tom Shisler, who worked as a financial planner at the North Pointe Financial Group in Akron, Ohio. He and his wife, Nora, had planned a weeklong vacation to Florida in early April with their two young children, Matt, age seven, and Gretchen, eighteen months. Matt was in the first grade at Silver Lake Elementary School and had a week off for Spring Break. It had been a long, cold winter, and Tom and Nora were eager to leave their home in Silver Lake Village, Ohio, and head south to warmer weather in the Sunshine State.

Tom, Nora, and the kids first headed to Palm Harbor, Florida, a charming community on the west coast in the Tampa Bay area, where they visited Tom's mother, who was recuperating from surgery for lung cancer. After a few relaxing days in Palm Harbor, they hopped in the car and made the two-hour drive to Disney World in Orlando. Tom and Nora were grateful for the sunshine and warmth and looked forward to spending the rest of the week with the kids at Magic Kingdom.

The weather was perfect, and it was a wonderful vacation for everyone. But Tom and Nora noted that there was something unusual going on with Matt. Each morning, he woke up with a pretty bad headache that was followed by copious vomiting. One morning, while the family was in the hotel restaurant having breakfast, the Disney characters—including Mickey, Minnie, and Goofy—came to visit them at their table, only to have Matt throw up over everyone. Then, and each day that followed, after the vomiting stopped, Matt's headache resolved over about an hour, and he felt much better. In fact, he felt so much better that he was able to accompany his family on all the rides and activities at Disney World and was back to his old self, as if nothing unusual had happened. But the headache and vomiting continued every morning.

Nora thought that was a little strange, but she wasn't too concerned because Matt looked so good for the rest of the day. And before they went on the trip, she had taken Matt and Gretchen to the pediatrician for a routine checkup. Their usual pediatrician, Dr. Steve Johnson, was on vacation at the time, so they saw someone else in the group. But both kids had a clean bill of health and seemed perfectly fine.

The family went back to Ohio over the weekend, and initially, Matt seemed to be doing okay. But during the next week, he started getting headaches at school. He reported this to his teacher, Mrs. Smith, who sent him to the nurse for Tylenol. Then on Friday, when he was scheduled to perform in the school play, he felt sick and vomited again. Nora knew that something was wrong and took him home to rest. She thought he might have a gastrointestinal bug.

On Sunday, Matt was scheduled to play in a basketball league game at the YMCA. But he said he didn't feel well and started to cry. He didn't want to play in the game. He couldn't give a reason. Nora wasn't sure what was going on. She suggested that Matt take a nap, which he did. After the nap, he felt better and sat down in the sunroom to watch television with his dad.

They were watching *The Flintstones*, a cartoon show, when Matt turned to his dad and asked, "Why are there two Freds on the screen?" Tom assured him there weren't two Freds and confirmed that by having Matt cover one eye at a time. Looking with either eye alone, Matt saw only one Fred. Tom explained what was going on to Nora, who by now realized that something might be seriously wrong. "It was a mother's intuition," she said.

Nora was worried but still hoped there might be a simple solution. Maybe Matt just needed a prescription for glasses. The next morning, she called her pediatrician, Dr. Johnson, who advised her to have Matt see the ophthalmologist Dr. Charles Davis of the Davis Eye Center in Cuyahoga Falls, Ohio. She set up an appointment for Matt to see Dr. Davis the following day.

So, on Tuesday, April 13, at 2 p.m., Nora brought Matt to see Dr. Davis in his office. Davis examined Matt and then left the room for fifteen minutes. He returned with a poker-faced expression.

"What's going on?" Nora asked.

"I'm not certain," Davis said. "I just talked to a buddy of mine, Dr. Robert Burnstine. He's a highly regarded pediatric ophthalmologist. He specializes in disorders of kids. I'd like you to see him. I think he'll be able to figure this out."

"Okay," Nora said, "I'll make an appointment."

"Not necessary, Nora," Dr. Davis said. "I've already made an appointment for you with him. He'll see you in his office at Akron Children's Hospital at 3 p.m. today."

Nora thanked him and headed off to see Dr. Burnstine. At this point, Nora had no idea what was to come. It made good sense to her that Matt would see a pediatric ophthalmologist. She didn't even question why the appointment had already been made by Dr. Davis to occur within the hour.

Dr. Robert "Boomer" Burnstine was indeed a highly regarded pediatric ophthalmologist. Burnstine met with Matt and found papilledema on fundoscopic exam, elevation of the optic discs, suggestive of increased intracranial pressure. He also found diplopia (double vision) from a right abducens nerve palsy, dysfunction of the sixth cranial nerve, the longest cranial nerve in the head, which acts to abduct the eye, moving it laterally. Matt's right eye was turned in. This finding also suggested increased intracranial pressure.

"I think he may have a brain tumor," he told Nora. "I want to get an MRI of his brain. I think you should call your husband and have him meet you here."

Nora began to cry, something she would do daily over the next several weeks. She tried to hide her tears from Matt, who was sitting beside her. It was later in the afternoon, and the MRI technicians were leaving the hospital, but Burnstine managed to convince them to stay to do the study. Nora called Tom, who came over immediately and met them in the MRI suite.

The scan took about an hour. It was performed before and after the administration of gadolinium, a rare-earth paramagnetic intravenous contrast agent that often helps light up various types of tumors. Matt was lying on the MRI table during the study while a group of doctors gathered around the computer monitor in the control room outside the scanner. Nora stood outside the control room, with tears streaming down her cheeks as she watched the group of doctors talking with one another and shaking their heads.

Dr. Burnstine spoke with Dr. Johnson, the family's pediatrician, on the phone and then called Nora in the MRI suite waiting room. He told her that Matt had a large brain tumor—the largest brain tumor they had ever seen at Akron Children's Hospital. Shaking with fear, Nora had only one question for Burnstine: "Is he going to live?"

"I don't know," Burnstine replied.

At the same time, Dr. Johnson called the MRI waiting room and spoke to Tom. Dr. Johnson had already called me and told me the story. We had decided to bring Matt to the emergency room at Rainbow Babies and Children's Hospital. Dr. Johnson told Tom about the tumor and the plan. Dr. Johnson, who was in his fifties, told Tom that this was only the second brain tumor he had ever seen in his entire career. Curiously, the only other time he'd seen a child with a brain tumor was earlier in the same week.

In the overall scheme of things, childhood brain tumors are relatively rare. That's one of the reasons their diagnosis can be elusive. Many of the presenting symptoms (headache, nausea, vomiting) are non-specific and occur more frequently with other common disorders, such as gastrointestinal disease and migraine. And because pediatric brain tumors are so rare, many pediatricians see only one or two cases in their entire careers—and some don't see any.

Tom was frightened, and Nora was panic-stricken, afraid to even look at Matt for fear he would see how scared she was. Nora remembers vividly how she felt. She became physically sick. She recalled that recently Matt had lost interest in playing basketball.

Thinking back, she could now see how frail he had become over the past several weeks, how thin his arms and legs were. She thought about the pain he must have been going through, what he must have endured. She remembered a recent picture he had drawn of himself in which he colored his eyes red. She thought, How could I have missed that? How did I not realize the suffering he must have been experiencing?

She blamed herself—something parents in this kind of situation often do, even though she had done nothing wrong.

"I tried to hold it together for Matt," she said. "But my mind was racing all over. Thinking about death, beyond sadness, shock. You ask for prayers like crazy. I wanted to hug Matt every second I could. It was like a bad dream."

Tom was teary-eyed, wondering, What will I do without my son? He and Nora each tried to boost the other up. They were scared and confused. They didn't know if their son was going to survive. Meanwhile, Matt was feeling okay and didn't realize what all the fuss was about.

They were both at Akron Children's Hospital with two cars. So, Nora drove home to grab a toothbrush and a change of clothes while Tom took Matt up to the roof of the parking garage to watch the Akron Aeros play. He wanted to distract Matt, though most of the anxiety was felt by the parents, not the child. The Akron Aeros were a Minor League Baseball team, a Double-A affiliate of the Cleveland Indians, now known as the Cleveland Guardians, a professional American League baseball team. The roof of the parking garage had a great view of the stadium, which seats about 7,600 fans. Today, the Akron Aeros team no longer exists. In 2013, they changed their name to the Akron RubberDucks, in honor of Akron's history as the Rubber Capital of the World.

At about 7 p.m. that evening, Tom and Nora arrived with Matt at the Rainbow Babies and Children's Emergency Room, where I met them. Nora remembers what I was wearing—my OR clothes, a blue blazer, and clogs. "Designer scrubs," I told them. "I'm not a fashion slave like everyone else. In a few years when this goes mainstream, remember where you saw it first."

It was my attempt to lighten the mood. The anxiety level in the room was palpable. I was with my resident, Tina Rodrigue, who has an excellent rapport with patients and families and helped bring the temperature down.

We went over the history, examined Matt, and reviewed his MRI with the family. There was a massive brain tumor indeed. It was cystic and solid, located at the top of the cerebellum, compressing the brain, putting pressure on the brainstem, and causing herniation of the cerebellum inferiorly through the foramen magnum, the large opening at the base of the skull through which the brainstem connects with the spinal cord. The tumor demonstrated enhancement after the administration of intravenous contrast and caused non-communicating hydrocephalus, a backup of cerebrospinal fluid in the blocked cerebral ventricles. All of this created increased intracranial pressure. It looked to me like an astrocytoma, an intrinsic tumor arising from the astrocytes, the star-shaped supporting cells of the cerebellum.

It was a dramatic scan. Matt would require surgery to remove the tumor. I outlined the plan, discussed the risks and benefits of the procedure, and obtained informed consent from Tom and Nora. We sent off some bloodwork, admitted Matt to the PICU, and placed him on intravenous dexamethasone to reduce the edema around the tumor and bring down the intracranial pressure. Nora would sleep on a couch in Matt's PICU room, and Tom would sleep in another room down the hall. Everything had happened so fast that day that it was hard for them to process what was going on.

I left the family and went off to do an emergency case in the OR. Several hours later, at about 1 a.m., as I was leaving to go home, I spotted Tom and Nora sitting in the hospital cafeteria atrium. The place was dark, and the cafeteria was closed. No one else was around. They had bought some food from a vending machine and were trying to understand what was going on with their young boy. I sat down with them for a few minutes. They were exhausted.

Tom told me it was the worst day of their entire lives. Nora told me she was running purely on adrenaline. This was their son. They didn't know if he would survive the surgery. "You don't know what to expect," she said. "You want to do everything you can to help your child, but this is uncharted territory." And if he survived, would he be the same kid he was before? Tom told me Matt was a very special kid—kind, gentle, and adored by everyone around him.

I tried to calm them down. Nora asked me repeatedly if Matt was going to live. "He has to live," she said repeatedly. Tom asked, "What am I ever gonna do without my little buddy?"

I told them we would make sure Matt would live. I told them I could imagine how scared they were—I was a parent too. I reassured them that we would do our best to get Matt through the surgery, that this was something we did all the time, like an auto mechanic changing the carburetor on a car. Realistically, I didn't tell them that I was scared too. This was one of the largest tumors I had ever seen.

They were well aware of all the surgical risks, and I didn't want to add to their anxiety. There was no way to handle the problem other than surgery. I tried to project confidence when I left them for the night. Nobody wants to hand over their child to a nervous surgeon. It's the delicate balance between honesty and hope. And hope is what keeps us all going in times of trouble. Where there is life, there is hope.

Meanwhile, Matt was resting comfortably in the PICU, except for the hourly wake-ups when the nurses checked his vital signs. The room where Tom slept was cold. He had a fitful night and was awake most of the time. Nora didn't sleep well either.

We operated on Matt on Wednesday, April 14, 1999. He awakened early that morning in good spirits. As a seven-year-old first-grader, he was too young to understand the gravity of what was to come. We told him we were going to surgery to remove a swelling from his head. Tom and Nora told him we would shave his head for the procedure, and that would make him look like his hero, Michael Jordan of the Chicago Bulls. It didn't hurt that the hospital had a life-size cardboard stand-up figure of Michael Jordan in the hallway that Matt really liked. Matt was cool as a cucumber as he was wheeled to the OR.

Nora accompanied Matt to the OR. She was terrified but made sure to put on a strong face for her son. He brought his prized three-foot-tall stuffed Sesame Street character, Ernie, with him into surgery, and we promised to perform the same procedure on Ernie. Nora left the OR, continuing to turn back over her shoulder to get a last glimpse of Matt as he was being intubated for general anesthesia, terrified about what lay ahead.

I performed the surgery with Ali Najafi, a very bright senior resident. First, we placed a right frontal burr hole and inserted a soft catheter into Matt's lateral cerebral ventricle to reduce the intracranial pressure by draining cerebrospinal fluid into a sterile bag. This would enable us to perform a posterior fossa craniotomy at the base of Matt's skull more safely and remove the tumor without fear of the brain herniating out of the head from the pressure of hydrocephalus.

To perform the posterior fossa craniotomy, we placed Matt in the sitting position. For this, the back of the OR bed is slowly raised bolt upright and the patient's head is fixed in a holder with the neck in moderate flexion. The advantage of this position for Matt's surgery is that his tumor was situated in the posterior fossa at the top of the cerebellum, just beneath the fibrous tentorium *(Latin- roof)* that separates the cerebellum from the overlying cerebral hemispheres. By sitting the patient upright, we can use gravity to help pull the cerebellum downward and give us some working room in the narrow corridor at the top of the cerebellum just beneath the fibrous tentorium. It also improves ventilation and reduces venous bleeding, which can sometimes be profuse.

But the sitting position is dangerous and comes with a cost. It cannot be utilized without an experienced anesthesiology team. Extensive monitoring is necessary to ensure safety of the patient. A major concern is the possibility of venous air embolism, a life-threatening condition in which air can enter the low pressure venous system or the non-collapsable venous sinuses and migrate to the right heart, causing hemodynamic instability, cardiovascular collapse, and, in some cases, paradoxical embolism to the brain, causing stroke. To monitor for venous air embolism, we placed a precordial doppler ultrasound probe on Matt's chest in front of the heart that allowed us to listen to high-frequency sound waves bouncing off his veins. We also inserted a central venous catheter and directed the tip into Matt's right cardiac atrium, confirming its position with a chest X-ray. This catheter would enable us to immediately aspirate air from the heart should an air embolism occur.

We made a midline incision in the back of Matt's head and removed a rectangular portion of his skull, with the top of the bone flap just underneath the two transverse sinuses—the large venous channels that ultimately return blood from the brain back to the heart. Then we opened the fibrous dura mater, exposing the cerebellum and the narrow working space on top of it, which we navigated using the operating microscope to resect the tumor.

We created a small opening in the top of the cerebellum and entered a tumor cyst, which we drained. This caused the brain to relax a bit more, enabling us to core out the tumor using an ultrasonic aspirator. It was a long, tedious dissection because the tumor was so large, but we were ultimately able to achieve a gross total resection of the tumor by enucleating it, coring it from the inside out, slowly marching forward until we reached the front of the tumor in the center of Matt's brain. We carefully dissected it off the large vein of Galen anteriorly at the depth of the exposure.

At this point, we had created a large hole at the top of the cerebellum where the tumor had been, and we had a spectacular view of the normal structures in the depths of the brain, including the vein of Galen, the internal cerebral veins, the basal veins of Rosenthal, and the back of the corpus callosum, the large bundle of white matter fibers that connects the two cerebral hemispheres. This infratentorial supracerebellar approach in the sitting position is demanding on the surgeon and the patient, but it provides the operator looking through the microscope with an extraordinary view of the magnificence of the anatomy at the center of the human brain.

We closed the dura sewing in a fibrous graft to prevent future compression of the cerebellum, replaced the bone flap, and sewed up the wound in layers, including the subcutaneous tissue and scalp, with absorbable sutures that don't have to be removed. The frozen section we sent to the pathologist came back as astrocytoma, low-grade. That was good news. We sent more tissue for special stains to better characterize the tumor. The anesthesia team extubated Matt on the OR table, and he woke up and was able to move all his extremities and follow commands. The operation lasted eleven hours, and we were all exhausted at the end.

The sitting position is particularly hard on the surgeon's arms, which have to be held up in the air and extended for long periods. I reminded the team that things could have been worse. The first documented sitting-position procedure was done in 1913 by Fedor Krause in Berlin, Germany, to remove a pineal region tumor in the center of the brain. He had poor illumination, no microscope, no microinstruments, no monitoring equipment, and no specialized head holder. The patient's head was held by an assistant for the duration of the operation. The operation we did was daunting for me in the best possible circumstances. I can't imagine what it must have been like for Krause and the neurosurgical pioneers operating over a century ago.

Tom and Nora had endured an excruciating time in the waiting room. The circulating nurse in our OR called them with updates every two hours. They tried to distract themselves. They had family with them. They read magazines, watched TV, and watched the clock. Nora kept thinking, What are they doing in there? What's taking so long? Just let me see my son. Please let him live.

Tom and Nora caught a glimpse of Matt as we wheeled him from the OR back to the PICU. His head was sore after the long operation, and he was crying from some incisional pain. Nora told me later it was the happiest sound she'd ever heard because she knew Matt was alive. After we settled him in the PICU, I met with the family. I told them we were able to get the whole tumor out, and it looked low-grade, that is, not cancer. Nora cried. We all went to the bedside. Matt was awake but had incisional pain. We gave him some intravenous analgesic medication and let Tom and Nora visit with him. The next morning, the postoperative MRI confirmed total resection of the tumor. That post-op MRI is the final exam for the neurosurgeon, ensuring that the surgical goals were reached and the brain was not injured. The final pathology returned two days later as pilocytic astrocytoma, WHO grade 1, a benign tumor. We all exhaled deeply.

The cerebellum (Latin for "little brain") is a diminutive term for cerebrum, the largest part of the brain. The bilobed cerebrum controls thought, consciousness, and other functions, including behavior, language, motor, and sensory activities. The cerebellum accounts for about 10 percent of the brain substance and sits posteriorly and inferiorly, beneath the temporal and occipital lobes of the cerebrum. The cerebellum controls balance and coordinates movement.

Matt's tumor arose from the superior aspect of his cerebellum at the top of the two cerebellar hemispheres and the midline cerebellar vermis (Latin for "worm") that bridges them. Because the tumor was so large, it compressed the cerebellar structures and caused swelling that was present for some time even after the tumor was removed. For that reason, it took a few days for Matt to get up and about, but he was young and resilient, and with physical and occupational therapy, he began walking up and down the hallway with assistance, making gains each day, and started doing stairs. He was discharged home after a week. The nursing team wheeled him to the door, and everyone watched and cheered as he walked unassisted to the car. The hospital staff gave him a gift to keep—the life-size cardboard poster of his hero, Michael Jordan.

When Matt got home, he was surprised to see a crowd of thirty people waiting for him in his driveway. He got applause when he got out of the car. There was a chalk message on the sidewalk that said "Welcome Home Matt." He was only seven years old and didn't really understand why all the people were there. What was all the fuss for? Matt didn't complain, however, about all the attention he continued to receive. And he got plenty of gifts, which came from his parents, neighbors, and dad's coworkers, and included state-of-the-art video games, such as Game Boy Color, Pokémon, Nintendo 64, and Mario Kart. It was a seven-year-old boy's dream come true.

Tom and Nora were still traumatized, still trying to process what they had been through. A few days after Matt was home, Nora had driven with both her kids to Marc's Grocery Market in Stow, Ohio. When she came out to drive home, she realized that she'd locked the keys inside the car. Fortunately, she had both kids with her, and eighteen-month-old Gretchen was in her arms, and everyone was safe. But she became hysterical and started bawling inconsolably. She still had lingering stress from Matt's recent hospitalization—he'd only been home for a few days.

There were no cell phones at the time, but a kind stranger went into the store and had the manager call the police. An officer arrived in a few minutes, looked at Nora, and wondered why she was so upset. After all, all she had done was lock her keys in the car. No one was injured. Everyone was okay. He asked Nora, "Is there something else going on in your life, ma'am? Is there anything you want to talk about?"

"Yes, officer, there sure is," she said, and proceeded to tell him in exquisite detail the whole saga she and her family had been going through, still sobbing the entire time.

The kind officer brought Nora and her kids to his squad car and let them sit inside while he retrieved the keys. He offered to accompany them home, but by now, Nora had composed herself, thanked the officer, and went on her way. But emotional episodes like this would continue to haunt her.

Matt made great strides and improved daily at home. For a while, he was eating like a horse, likely because of the steroids he'd been on perioperatively. Kids often do surprisingly well once they get out of the hospital and return to their familiar surroundings at home. His walking returned to normal after a few weeks. He was homeschooled for the next few months to complete first grade and returned to in-person classes in the fall to begin second grade with his peers. He was back to his old self.

But something was different in the classroom. Why are all the kids acting so weird? he thought. These are my friends. They don't want to get close to me. They're acting as if they're afraid of me. I'm the same guy I always was.

And that's exactly what was happening. The kids looked at the scar on the back of his head and were afraid they would catch what he had. But over time, the anxiety abated, and by the end of the year, Matt was accepted as a member of the group, just as he'd been before.

Recently, Matt shared an anecdote with me that I had not previously been aware of. In January 2000, ten months after Matt's surgery, I was holding a birthday celebration at the hospital for Elvis Presley, who would have been sixty-five years old at the time. We dressed up and had a karaoke session in which several of my patients and I sang, danced, and put on a show for the kids who were hospitalized and their families. Matt joined us and was out there on the stage, having the time of his life.

He had told his teacher he had to go to the hospital to get an MRI, which clearly was not the case. Oops. I guess that may make me an accomplice to the corruption of a minor. Although I feel I must have some guilt by association, I hope I will be forgiven. After all, wasn't this part of the healing process? I will argue that it surely was. In any event, I'm hoping the episode will be forgotten because it happened a quarter century ago, which must be well beyond the statute of limitations.

I have followed Matt over the years with serial surveillance MRIs, which, fortunately, have shown no evidence of residual or recurrent tumor. It took him a couple of years to really realize the gravity of what he had gone through. It became clear to him by the time he was in the fourth grade. As he grew up, he became a serious advocate for children's health. Even when he was just thirteen years old in the seventh grade, Matt traveled with his family to Washington, DC, along with the National Association of Children's Hospitals and Related Institutions (NACHRI) to lobby Congress for a multimillion-dollar bill to provide more funding to help train specialists. They were successful in their efforts.

Matt was voted Student of the Year in eighth grade. He went on to graduate from Cuyahoga Falls High School, where he won the Perseverance Award for overcoming obstacles and not giving up. In college, at the University of Akron, he majored in communications and was on the Dean's List. He played tuba in the marching band, the same instrument his dad had played in college at the University of Iowa. The apple doesn't fall far from the tree. Matt's younger sister, Gretchen, who was just eighteen months old at the time of his surgery, graduated from Ohio State

University and works as the social media manager for Condado Restaurants. She lives in Columbus, Ohio.

Matt lives in Cincinnati, Ohio, where he is now the national director of digital marketing for King's Hammer FC, a pre-professional soccer club. The scrawny little kid he was in first grade now stands six feet four inches tall, an inch taller than his dad. His wife, Jane, works as a special education teacher. She graduated from the University of Cincinnati. They met on a dating app in 2019 and married in March 2022.

Many years have passed since April 14, 1999, the day when Matt had his surgery and his family's lives were turned upside down. He thinks back about it often and remembers having gone through the ordeal as a seven-year-old boy in a state of blissful oblivion. Now, as an adult, he has a much more sober view of what transpired. Random events trigger his memory and bring him back to the time of surgery as if it were yesterday. He gets emotional at times, thinking about what life would have been like if things had turned out differently.

"It affects my wife Jane, too," he said. "Sometimes she gets overcome with emotion and wells up. She once told me she didn't know what life would be like without me. I told her not to worry; that was something she'd never have to worry about."

"It puts life in perspective for me," Matt said. "It changed me as a person. Little things that might get someone upset don't matter to me. I'm a glass-is-half-full guy now. I'm happy to be alive. Now that I'm older and thinking about having kids of my own, I wonder how I'd react if my child were to have a brain tumor. I would definitely be a basket case." Matt did comment that he hopes that someday his child would grow up to play the tuba in the marching band. "We need to make sure the tuba thing makes it into the third generation," he said.

Many are familiar with the proverb, "Time heals all wounds." It is attributed to the ancient Greek poet, Menander, who lived around 300 BC. His actual words were, "Time is the healer of all necessary evils." Menander was a wise man who made that observation more than two millennia ago. And indeed, the passage of time can be effective in mitigating the pain of many types of traumas. Time heals, for sure. There are some wounds, however, that never heal. Other wounds have a persisting effect and heal only partially with time.

The diagnosis of a pediatric brain tumor is a life-changing event. It has a lasting impact, not only on the patient, but on the entire family. This is true for Matt's family, even though the story has a happy ending—the tumor was benign and has not come back. In spite of this, Nora continues to get flashbacks from time to time. She sometimes breaks down unexpectedly when talking with friends. Her thoughts go back to the day when she first saw the large brain tumor on Matt's MRI. "Every time I look at him, even now, I say thank God, I have him," she said. "And I might not have. We were the lucky ones. My heart goes out to families whose outcome was not so fortunate."

Tom Shisler is a strong man, but he, too, still feels the lingering effects of the trauma his family went through so many years ago. He remembers hosting the rehearsal dinner the night before Matt's wedding. It's customary for the groom's father to get up and make a toast. Tom became very emotional and gave a gripping, heartfelt speech about what his very special son had gone through as a young boy. Matt had never seen his father cry before. Many in the room were hearing the story for the first time. Tom noted that at one point, he wasn't sure which way things were heading. He didn't even know if Matt would be alive to celebrate a night like this. He brought the entire room to tears.

Matt is now grown up, married, and out of the house, living in a different city. Tom thinks of him every day. Each morning when Tom wakes up, he has a ritual in which he brushes his teeth and walks into Matt's room. The room has become a shrine to Matt's life, a celebration of all that he accomplished while growing up. The life-size cardboard cutout of Michael Jordan is there, along with all of Matt's awards, his Dean's List certificates, his large stuffed Ernie, a photo of him and his friends and one of him with me in my office, the name tag he wore when he went as a child to lobby Congress in Washington, and memorabilia from his tuba days in the marching band. Tom, Nora, and Matt remain very close and speak on the phone at least once or twice every day. Matt's childhood ordeal has brought them closer. The lingering effects of trauma cannot be overstated.

Rose Kennedy, the mother of former President JFK and matriarch of the Kennedy family, endured more than her share of trauma during her lifetime. Her thoughtful reflection is powerful:

"It has been said that time heals all wounds. I don't agree. The wounds remain. In time, the mind, protecting its sanity, covers them with scar tissue, and the pain lessens, but is never gone."

CHAPTER 5

Perseverance

"Our greatest weakness lies in giving up. The most certain way to succeed is always to try just one more time."

THOMAS ALVA EDISON

The first thing I noticed about little Gracie was her sadness. The edges of her mouth were turned downward, and her cheeks hung low as she sat motionless, looking straight ahead with a blank stare. Her parents, Carla and Bruce Tucker, had brought her to see me at Boston Children's Hospital in late July of 2013 because of an abnormality noted on an MRI of her brain performed the day before. They had traveled from another state and were tired from the trip. But just a brief glance at Gracie across the room made it clear that she was more than just tired. There was something serious going on.

Grace was two-and-a-half years old. She was born by cesarean section at thirty-two weeks of gestation (eight weeks prematurely) following an uncomplicated pregnancy. She was a dizygotic (fraternal) twin, meaning that there were two separate eggs fertilized by two separate sperm. Grace was twin B, with a birth weight of only three pounds, twelve ounces. Her sister Emma, who came out first, was twin A.

Carla brought her twin infant girls home from the hospital and watched them develop normally. But when Grace was a little more than two years old, about three months before I met her, she began to change. The change was subtle at first, but Carla realized that things were a little off. Grace seemed more tired during the daytime and began spitting up her food frequently. She became more irritable. Her hands became tremulous, and she had trouble with coordination. She started tipping her head back, and her gait became unsteady. Carla thought she was walking like a drunk person.

As time went on, Carla became more concerned and brought Grace to see the pediatrician. But what was obvious to Carla was not so obvious to others. Grace didn't look so bad at the pediatrician's office. It wasn't clear what was going on. The decision was made to follow a course of watchful waiting.

Over the next month, things got progressively worse. Grace began slurring her words. She became weak in her arms and legs. Her gait became more unsteady. She held her mouth open and began gagging. The vomiting, which initially occurred about once a week, became more frequent. She had lost four pounds in two months. Carla became more concerned and brought Grace to see the doctor a total of four times over a three-month period. The doctors thought something was wrong but weren't sure what was going on. Was she hypothyroid? They ran thyroid tests that came back normal. They thought it might be a gastrointestinal virus or something else and continued to wait and see if she would improve. They set up an appointment for Grace to see a specialist at the medical center in several weeks. Carla was frustrated and angry. She knew there was something very wrong with her daughter, and she couldn't understand why she was sent home from the doctor's office each time without a diagnosis or treatment plan.

Grace's deterioration continued. Carla thought she began to look like a zombie. Her face was expressionless and didn't move. She became sleepier. Carla worked as an investigative social worker for the Department of Child Protective Services, and Bruce worked as a route sales deliveryman for a bread company, so neither was home during most days. Grace and her sister, Emma, would spend most of the time with their grandmother, Sharon, who watched over them religiously at her own home nearby. One day, Sharon noticed that Grace's walking was so wobbly that she kept bumping into the walls. Grace had been eating poorly and could barely even swallow soft food. Sharon found her lying on the couch, drooling. Then she vomited profusely all over the couch. From across the room, Sharon overheard Grace talking to herself: "You're gonna be okay. You're not gonna die."

That was it. Sharon lost it. She had reached her breaking point. She called her daughter at work.

"Carla," she said, "she's much worse. Something very bad is going on. I can't do this anymore. I am not going to be the one to sit here and watch her die."

Carla left work immediately and raced over to pick up Grace and take her to the nearest medical center, which was still about an hour away. Carla was terrified as she told the story to the ER docs, who saw that Grace was lethargic. But they didn't think things were as bad as Carla made them seem. They asked if Grace could have overdosed on medication, even though Carla had not given her any medication and didn't have any medication in the home. They questioned Carla in a manner that made her feel as if they were accusing her of drugging her daughter. They asked if Carla had left open vials of medication near Grace.

Carla felt humiliated, particularly because it was her job to investigate cases of child maltreatment and abuse for the state. The ER docs sent Grace home with plans to come back in a couple of weeks for the elective outpatient visit that had already been set up weeks earlier by her local pediatrician. Carla left disheartened, feeling as if the doctors thought she was fabricating her daughter's illness, a syndrome sometimes called Munchausen by proxy. The name originally comes from the fictional German nobleman, Baron Munchausen, who was known for his dramatic but fabricated stories. The current classification is now called "factitious disorder imposed on another."

It was a disorder that Carla did not have. The next day, she recounted her story to a friend, who looked at Grace and knew instantly that something serious was going on. It turns out that her friend's child had been diagnosed with a brain tumor a few years ago, with a presentation like Grace's. Her friend took it upon herself to make an appointment for Grace to be seen the following day at Boston Children's Hospital. She joined Carla and Grace for the three-hour bus ride and visit. Grace was seen by a neurologist who was concerned by her exam, ordered a stat MRI of her brain, and referred her to me.

With that background, I got up from my chair to examine little Gracie, who was sitting on her dad's lap across from me in my office. She was pale and rail thin. Her eyes were partially open, and she was awake but appeared to be dazed, with no interest in what was going on in the room. She was minimally verbal and spoke in a soft nasal voice. Her eyes were pointed straight ahead with limitation of abduction bilaterally, that is, she couldn't move either eye to the side when she looked either to the right or left. She had a facial diplegia, with marked weakness of the facial muscles on both sides, explaining her droopy cheeks and sad appearance. She was drooling from the sides of her mouth. She had diffuse weakness of her arms and legs, with low muscle tone. She could ambulate only with a lot of assistance, with her feet wide apart in a slow, unsteady gait.

Grace's MRI was striking. There was a large intrinsic tumor filling her brainstem, the "command central" part of the brain that keeps us alive. The tumor was situated at the junction of the pons and medulla and appeared to fill the entire brainstem at that level, extending exophytically outside the front of the brainstem with only a very thin rim of normal brainstem tissue behind it. I had never seen anything like this in my life. I stared at the scan, bewildered, wondering how the approximately one billion neurons traversing the brainstem could pass through the paper-thin rim of remaining tissue at the back end of the mass. I wondered how anyone with a tumor this large and in this location could even be alive.

Then I composed myself and tried as best I could to appear calm, competent, and experienced so that I could provide some comfort to the family. I brought Carla and Bruce behind my desk to show them the MRI on my computer. "Wow, that's one whopping tumor," I said, wondering why I chose those particular words as I heard them coming out of my mouth. That was probably not the most consoling way to break the news, but I suspect I was still unsettled by the massive size of the brainstem tumor I was seeing for the first time. "And it's sitting in a pretty significant part of the brain. We now have the explanation for what's been going on these past few months."

The tumor was not subtle. Carla and Bruce were overcome by relief that we had found the problem but were fearful about what could be done about it. I told them we were going to have to operate to find out what the tumor was and to remove as much as we safely could.

"The operation will be tricky," I said, "because the tumor is sitting right smack in the center of some important real estate. This is the part of the brain that keeps us alive, keeps us conscious, lets us move our eyes, face, and limbs, tells our heart to beat, and allows us to breathe, speak, and swallow. There is a silver lining though. I don't think this is cancer. I can't be certain, but I think the tumor is going to be benign. It's just in a very dangerous location."

I don't routinely tell the family whether I think the tumor is benign or malignant before surgery, because there's no way to know for certain. If the tumor has features on imaging studies that make it look malignant and it turns out to be benign at surgery, then everyone breathes a deep sigh of relief. But if the tumor appears to be benign on the MRI and then comes back malignant at surgery, that's a much more unpleasant conversation, and one that I try to preempt. But I had developed a good rapport with Carla and Bruce, and I try as best I can to be honest with families without taking away hope. After all this family had been through, I felt it was important to bring some hope into the discussion.

The imaging characteristics on the different sequences of the MRI and its geometry, location, patchy enhancement following the administration of intravenous gadolinium contrast material, and significant restriction of diffusion suggested that this was likely an epidermoid (skin-like) tumor. An epidermoid is a benign tumor. In this case, it was likely that the tumor was present before

Grace was even born. Because it started early during embryonic development, it likely displaced the normal neurons of the brainstem, pushing them away and allowing them to grow around it. There are other, more lethal brainstem tumors, such as the diffuse intrinsic pontine glioma (DIPG), recently renamed diffuse midline glioma (DMG), that intermingle with the normal nerve fibers as they grow, making them unresectable and one of the most lethal tumors in the nervous system.

I went on to have a detailed discussion with Carla and Bruce about plans. I would send Grace for more high-resolution MRI studies. I discussed the different surgical corridors for approaching this tumor and told them I wanted to go over the plans with some of my expert colleagues across the country, because this was such an unusual case. I was candid and let them know that I had never removed a tumor this large in this location, but that we had a lot of specialized equipment to help make the surgery safer. Carla and Bruce asked a few more questions and left nervously, saying they were appreciative of my honesty. I would mobilize our team and set up surgery. Later, Carla told me she was in a state of shock. Things were happening so quickly that she didn't have time to properly process what was going on. She said it felt like an out-of-body experience.

We do indeed have lots of equipment to help make surgery safer. Unfortunately, technology is an adjunct, but it isn't the solution. We all knew this would be a hazardous operation with high risks. Particularly in a complex case like this, surgical judgment is all-important. That's why I decided to consult with other experts before going to the OR.

Not surprisingly, I got a wide variety of opinions. One neurosurgeon recommended that I operate transorally, through the mouth, because the tumor had broken through the brainstem anteriorly. This afforded the advantage of gaining access to the tumor without having to transgress any of the normal brainstem tissue. But the disadvantage was that it would be a challenging approach through a long, narrow corridor that would communicate the oral cavity, along with all of its intrinsic bacterial flora, with the intradural compartment, creating the risk of an infection, such as meningitis or a brain abscess.

Another senior neurosurgeon recommended an anterolateral approach at the base of the skull, which avoided the need to go through the mouth but would still permit access to the front of the tumor that had broken through the brainstem anteriorly. The disadvantage of this approach was that coming from the side, I would have to work adjacent to many unforgiving cranial nerves innervating movement of the eyes and face and swallowing, and although I would see the front of the tumor, I would still be coming from the side and would have to work around the corner to remove it, without good visualization.

Another colleague suggested treating Grace with upfront radiation therapy to eliminate altogether the risks of surgery, which would be high. This is an approach that we sometimes use for palliative care when the tumor appears highly malignant and inoperable, as is the case with some diffuse midline gliomas. But in the modern era, it is rare for us to treat without a tissue diagnosis, especially now that we are able to identify molecular mutations in tumors that can potentially be targeted with personalized designer drugs. But the main reason I rejected this plan was because I believed Grace's tumor was likely an epidermoid, a benign "skin-like" neoplasm that would not respond to radiation. And radiating the brainstem is something not to be taken lightly, as it is associated with significant short- and long-term risks.

Ultimately, I decided to use a standard midline posterior approach working through the floor of the fourth ventricle at the base of the brain. This would provide good access to the back of the brainstem in order to reach the tumor. There are articles written about safe approaches to enter the brainstem that can avoid injury to essential cranial nerve nuclei. In my opinion, there are no safe entry zones to the brainstem because of the interconnectedness of all these important neuronal structures. It's just that some entry zones are safer than others.

I chose to enter the brainstem in the midline from behind, knowing that we would be working right between the bilateral paired sixth (abducens) and seventh (facial) cranial nerve nuclei, which are situated right next to each other. The reason I chose this route is that I knew these nuclei were already impaired. Grace could not abduct her eyes (move them laterally) because of dysfunction of the sixth cranial nerves, and she could not move either side of her face because of impairment of the adjacent seventh cranial nerves. Since these cranial nerves were already not working, I felt I really couldn't make them worse. And if I could stay in the midline, I would only have to go through a paper-thin region of the brainstem before reaching the tumor, thereby causing a minimal amount of brain-tissue disruption.

So, we set out to do the surgery early in the morning on Thursday, August 8, 2013. I did the case in the MR-OR with two extraordinarily gifted assistants, Scellig Stone and Brad Gross. The MR-OR is an impressive high-tech suite in which we can do the operation and stop the case along the way with the patient's head open, roll an MRI scanner out of an adjacent "garage," and take some pictures. Operating in the MR-OR suite is not without risk and takes some careful planning. Everyone on the staff has to undergo specialized training. Nothing that is magnetized can be in the room. The magnet in the scanner has such a strong force that it can suddenly pull objects toward it, which could result in injury or even death to the patient.

But the intraoperative MRI (iMRI) can be of great value. Maintaining sterile technique, we can image the brain to help guide the surgery. These images can offer information about the completeness of our surgical resection, letting us know if there might be a nubbin of tumor hiding around the corner that we couldn't see directly. The intraoperative MRI also gives us assurance that we haven't created any bleeding that we might not be able to see directly in the operative field. And an intraoperative scan at the end of the case can eliminate the need for a postoperative study in the radiology suite the following day, which can require sedation with anesthesia, particularly for young children like Gracie.

This was the most complex operation I had ever undertaken, and I made sure to use every adjunctive agent possible to enhance the safety of the procedure. In addition to the intraoperative MRI, we used image guidance with computer-based frameless stereotactic navigation, translating the two-dimensional anatomy of the preoperative MRI by computer into the three-dimensional space of the OR. This enabled us to use our surgical instruments sort of like magic wands so that we could touch any place on the head and identify the shortest and safest route to the tumor. We also used intraoperative electrophysiologic neuromonitoring, including motor-evoked potentials and somatosensory-evoked potentials, to assess function of the brainstem while Gracie was asleep, along with electrical leads to analyze the function of the lower cranial nerves seven to twelve bilaterally.

Gracie was positioned prone on the OR table, and we incised the back of her scalp in the midline and removed a piece of the occipital bone at the base of her skull, opened the dura, and worked under high magnification with guidance provided by a high-powered microscope. We used a telovelar approach, dividing thin membranes to open the cerebellomedullary fissure (the space between the cerebellum and the medulla of the lower brainstem) on each side. This enabled us to reflect the cerebellar hemispheres laterally using natural planes to provide us with a wide exposure of the fourth ventricle, the cerebrospinal fluid chamber that lies just behind the lower brainstem. Staring at the brainstem through the microscope, we could see the underlying tumor bulging up at us through a very thin translucent layer of normal brain tissue.

We made a small opening in the midline of the brainstem just inferior to the sixth and seventh cranial nerves, found the tumor, and removed it with great care. The tumor consisted of thick, milky-white, flaky material, and the pathology was as we had predicted: a benign epidermoid tumor. After resecting the tumor, we saw a glistening tumor capsule that was densely adherent to the surrounding brainstem. We resected a portion of this capsule but were careful not to tug too hard, as prior reports of similar surgeries described high rates of morbidity and mortality following aggressive manipulation of the tumor capsule when it was stuck to the brainstem. We confirmed gross total resection of the tumor by inserting a thin endoscope lens inside the resection cavity and finding clean margins circumferentially. An intraoperative MRI also showed no evidence of residual tumor. The brainstem had collapsed down to its normal size. The intraoperative neuromonitoring remained intact. We replaced Gracie's bone flap with titanium microplates and screws and sewed up her incision with absorbable sutures. Then we woke her up.

To our surprise and delight, Gracie made a remarkable recovery, much quicker and better than we would have ever predicted. It had been a long, tedious operation—Gracie was in the OR for the entire day. Carla and Bruce were worried that something had gone wrong because the operation took so long. But when they saw her standing up in her crib in the PICU, tears of happiness filled their eyes. She improved at a rapid pace every day and was discharged home after an uneventful week in the hospital.

When I saw her in a follow-up visit a month later, I almost didn't recognize her. She was another person. Her sensorium was brighter, and she could speak clearly. She was eating well and gaining weight. Her eyes now moved conjugately, and her facial weakness had disappeared completely. Her strength had improved, and she was walking independently and even dancing.

Carla and Bruce were ecstatic, and we were just as overjoyed, though somewhat flabbergasted. Grace's recovery seemed too good to be true. The brainstem is a challenging structure, and when we core out a tumor inside it, there are usually significant neurological sequelae that may remain for life—or take at least months before they improve. I suspect that we got lucky in that Grace's tumor had enlarged slowly and gradually compressed and displaced the important brainstem neurons and cranial nerve nuclei outward. Enucleating the tumor must have taken pressure off these structures, explaining why her eye movements, facial weakness, and gait got so much better. Scellig, Brad, and I walked around with a little extra bounce in our steps.

Sadly, our joy was short-lived. Two months after surgery, Carla called me to say that Gracie's appetite had worsened, and her walking had become unsteady again. Initially, I was in denial. I suspected that it might have been related to tapering off her steroids and that there might have been some residual brainstem edema causing the problem. So, we slowed down her steroid taper. But three months after surgery, she was no better. If anything, her walking was a little worse, and her face began drooping again. We repeated an MRI, which showed the return of the brainstem mass, almost to the same size as it was originally.

How could this happen? The tumor was an epidermoid. It was benign. Benign tumors don't come back once they are completely resected. And Grace's tumor was completely resected. And even if we had left a small piece of tumor that we couldn't see, which was unlikely, benign tumors don't recur this quickly. It didn't make sense. We had confirmed in the OR by direct microsurgical inspection and by MR imaging that we had removed the entire tumor. Could it have been an infection? Maybe an abscess had developed in the operative bed that was mimicking a recurrent tumor. We sent off bloodwork for inflammatory markers—CBC, ESR, CRP, and cultures. They were all normal. We did a lumbar puncture to analyze the cerebrospinal fluid for infection, but all tests came back normal. We were stymied.

Over the next month, Grace continued to worsen with lethargy, daily emesis, return of oculomotor and facial paralysis, diffuse weakness of the limbs, and gait unsteadiness. We were back at the starting gate. She was exactly as she was before we had operated on her. Carla and Bruce were scared. There was no question that something bad was going on. My premature exuberance after the successful surgery turned to confusion and sorrow. The tumor must have come back. There was no other alternative. Just months after a complex operation on Gracie's brainstem, I would have to admit failure and go back and reoperate.

And so back to the OR I went, along with my colleagues Scellig and Brad. And we did the identical surgery once again in the MR-OR suite, with all the elaborate surgical adjunctive measures we had used the first time. The thick, flaky, milky-white tumor had indeed recurred, and we carefully removed it again. We suspected that the recurrent epidermoid material was not the result of new cellular tumor growth but instead had been secreted by the residual capsule of the tumor that was adherent to the brainstem. Therefore, this time we chose to remove more of the tumor capsule. This was a dangerous maneuver, and we were aware of the high risk of complications related to peeling the capsule off the surrounding neural structures of the brainstem. But this capsule was what secreted the thick, milky tumor mass that came back, and we couldn't keep operating on Gracie every few months.

Under microsurgical and endoscopic guidance, we resected as much of the tumor capsule as we thought would be safe, even to the point at which Gracie became transiently hypertensive and bradycardic (slow heart rate) in the OR, signs of serious impending dysfunction. So, we stopped the resection at that point. But by now, we had removed the entire tumor, and most but not all of the tumor capsule. We were now able to look through the gaping hole we had created in the brainstem, from back all the way to the front. We had a breathtaking view that I had never seen before. We could now see right through the brainstem and visualize the large basilar and vertebral arteries, which sit in front, with virtually no brain tissue blocking our view. The normal residual brainstem tissue had become paper-thin from pressure and was pushed away to the sides. I marveled at the anatomy and at the wisdom of nature, wondering how these normal brainstem neurons could still function after being pushed outward into a razor-thin perimeter of tissue.

Once again, the intraoperative MRI confirmed total resection of the tumor, but this time, Grace's recovery was more complicated. She had a prolonged gaze palsy and prolonged significant bilateral facial weakness. Her voice was soft, and her speech was slurred the way it was before the first operation. She had difficulty swallowing and even required temporary placement of a gastrostomy feeding tube for nutrition. Her walking was unsteady, and she required long-term physical and occupational therapy. It was a long, tedious, difficult recovery. I believe the reason it took so long was that we had to manipulate the brainstem significantly in order to remove most of the capsule to prevent recurrence of the tumor and allow the normal cerebrospinal fluid to bathe through the operative bed.

But over the next several months, Gracie surprised us again and made an amazing recovery. Her gaze palsy and facial weakness resolved. Her smile returned. Her speech normalized. Her swallowing improved, and she began taking solid foods and liquids normally so that her feeding tube could be removed. Her balance returned, and after eight months, she was able to ambulate independently and could walk and run. It was a long haul, but it was worth the wait.

Over the years, I have remained close with the Tuckers, and I check in on Grace with phone calls and emails. She is now fifteen years old and is streamlined in regular classes in a public school, where she is doing well in most subjects but struggling somewhat with processing in math. She is a spunky kid with a lot of grit and passion. She loves animals and wants to be a veterinarian when she grows up.

Curiously, like some of my other young brain tumor patients who have emerged from the nightmares of treatment, she is terrified of going to school. And this scares her more than the treatment she had undergone for her brainstem tumor. I was surprised to hear this, because the Tuckers live in a small, cozy, rural village. But multiple times, Carla or Sharon have been called to bring Grace home because of school violence. It's stuff that I had never experienced when I was growing up. One kid threw a desk at the teacher. Another threw chairs and broke windows in the classroom. And apparently, such behavioral outbursts have been frequent. There were several shootings in buildings adjacent to the school, to the point that Carla has been considering homeschooling Gracie.

Carla sends me pictures and videos of Grace from time to time. Looking at her, you would have no idea what she had gone through as a young toddler. She has a broad, beautiful smile and plays with her cat, runs in the grass, and climbs trees. There is a charming video of her wearing a tutu, dancing flawlessly as a ballerina. It is gratifying that a decade after surgery, her clinical response has remained durable, and there's been no evidence of recurrent tumor on serial MRIs.

I've learned a lot caring for little Gracie. Intrinsic brainstem epidermoid tumors are extremely rare, histologically benign, and have been associated with a very high surgical morbidity and mortality because of their eloquent location. The first description of an epidermoid tumor was in 1829 by the French anatomist and pathologist, Jean Cruveilhier. He called it *tumeur perlée* (pearly tumor) because of its smooth, white, glistening appearance and its striking resemblance to mother of pearl. In 1945, the legendary neurosurgeon Walter Dandy of Johns Hopkins called epidermoids "perhaps the most beautiful tumors in the human body."

Epidermoid tumors are usually congenital, arising in the third to fifth weeks of embryological development due to an incomplete separation of neural tissue from the overlying skin. They can also arise later in life, acquired following surgery or trauma.

Gracie's epidermoid was certainly congenital. And rare. There have only been thirteen reported cases of brainstem epidermoids in the past twenty years. They appear to be the result of disordered embryogenesis and occur at a characteristic location at the pontomedullary junction, with the pons above and the medulla below. Although they appear to be intrinsic tumors and can occupy almost the entirety of the brainstem at the level at which they occur, these tumors actually behave as extrinsic masses that invaginate (fold back) into the developing brainstem. That's why we were able to remove the tumor without having to disrupt the normal surrounding brainstem neurons.

Epidermoid tumors contain an avascular capsule of squamous epithelial cells that secrete deposits of cheesy debris to form a mass. They usually grow slowly in a linear, non-exponential fashion. The growth of the mass was due to secretion of the cheesy semisolid debris from the tumor capsule, not from division of tumor cells themselves. That explains why Grace's tumor, which was benign, could regrow so soon after resection. Nevertheless, the growth was much quicker than usual. Normally, these tumors enlarge slowly over years.

The brainstem epidermoid is a good example of what can happen when a benign tumor occurs in a malignant location. The neurosurgical literature is replete with case examples of devastating outcomes following attempted resection of these tumors when the capsule is densely adherent to the important surrounding neurovascular structures. In the modern era, with all our high-tech adjuncts, including intraoperative MRI, frameless stereotactic navigation, electrophysiologic neuromonitoring, and endoscope-assisted microsurgical approaches, resection of these tricky brainstem epidermoids will likely be safer. But measured surgical judgment is as important, and arguably even more important, than all of these sophisticated technological advances. Surgical judgment is important in determining when to operate, when not to operate, how to find the safest surgical corridor, and when to stop the operation. In my mind, the optimal management of these challenging intrinsic brainstem epidermoid tumors remains conservative surgery with resection of as much of the tumor capsule as is safely possible.

But the main lesson I learned in caring for Gracie was not about surgical anatomy or surgical technique. It was about the importance of perseverance. Mother is always right. As a pediatric neurosurgeon, I take those words very seriously. Carla knew there was something very wrong with her daughter right from the start. A mother knows her child better than anyone, and she can pick up abnormalities that others might miss because she spends so much time with her child. Carla brought Gracie to see a series of doctors and health-care providers and was turned away every time. If she were not so doggedly persistent, Gracie would likely not be alive today. I also learned about the importance of perseverance for the surgeon. I had to swallow my pride after what I felt was a perfectly successful curative operation, admit defeat, and go back and operate again.

In the words of Ralph Waldo Emerson, "The greatest glory in living lies not in never failing, but in rising every time we fall."

CHAPTER 6

Star Gazer

"We have calcium in our bones, iron in our veins,
carbon in our souls, and nitrogen in our brains,
93% stardust, with souls made of flames, we
are all just stars that have people's names."

Nikita Gill
British Indian poet
"93% Stardust" from *Your Soul Is a River*, 2016

"I really like what you've done with the place. I think it brings the room together very nicely."

Those were Daniel Stinebring's first words when we met in my office many years ago. He was accompanied by his wife, Lynn Powell. It was Monday morning, May 10, 1999, and he had been referred to me by his primary care physician, Dr. Georgia Newman. Dan had been scanning the room, taking things in, and was clearly captivated by the two life-sized pink Elvis Presley lamps carefully situated, like twin towers, on each end of my desk. He appeared equally impressed by the velvet Elvis portrait on the wall and a Sigmund Freud action figure on the table nearby. Since he seemed interested, I took a moment to point out my prized possession, a framed piece of the waistband from a certified pair of Elvis's event-worn underwear. The certification came in the form of a faded, unsigned, mimeographed piece of paper.

"Those are all gifts," I said somewhat sheepishly. "It's crazy, I know. I keep them in here to lighten the mood. I'm a pediatric neurosurgeon, so I usually care for children. Also, my wife won't let me bring any of this stuff home."

As a forty-five-year-old man, Dan was considerably older than most of my patients at Rainbow Babies and Children's Hospital in Cleveland, Ohio. He was a genuinely pleasant guy with a relaxed, easygoing personality. But after talking with him for only a few minutes, it became clear to me that he was no ordinary individual. He was extremely smart. He became passionate and animated when he spoke about a variety of topics, including baseball, sailing, and politics. And his wife, Lynn, who took copious notes during the visit, was equally accomplished. But Dan was sent to see me not because of his age but because of his problem, which was unique.

"I'm an astrophysicist," he said nonchalantly. "And I've been seeing stars for the past few months."

Hmm, where are we going with this? I thought to myself. Was he really an astrophysicist? Was he making a joke? What's the punchline? Or was there a deeper meaning to his words?

In medicine, we place a great deal of emphasis on the chief complaint. Sometimes patients have multiple somatic issues, and it's easy to get sidetracked and lose sight of what brought them to see the doctor in the first place. Everything flows from the chief complaint—it enables the physician to focus on the rest of the history and examination and tailor what further tests might be indicated.

It turns out that Dan was indeed an astrophysicist. At first glance, his chief complaint didn't even sound like a complaint at all. Seeing stars. Isn't that what astrophysicists are supposed to do? Isn't that what draws them to the field? They go out in the darkness of night, gaze up at the heavens, and marvel at the splendor of the cosmos. Not a bad job.

The problem for Dan was that he was seeing stars in the daytime. And there was no telescope.

The first episode happened three months earlier. Dan was taking a shower, and the warm water was pouring down on his face. When he took his head out of the water stream, he saw stars, bright and dancing around, and the effect lasted for ten seconds or more. He thought, hmm, pretty cool, but what's causing *that!?*

Over the next several weeks, Dan continued to see stars and experience visual problems. As a skilled scientist, he kept a detailed journal, noting that the stars and afterimages of flashing lights would appear in the upper left part of his visual field, particularly when he would blink or move quickly from one scene to another. He astutely noted that the flashing lights were not just in one eye but both. They were in the left visual field. Sometimes he saw a crescent in the left lower part of his visual field. The stars often came on, along with dizziness, when he got up quickly. Afterimages sometimes persisted at a reduced level for up to a minute. When he rubbed his left eye, he felt a lingering afterimage of stars. Sometimes when he stood up quickly after sitting for a while, he described a "mini blackout" in his left visual field. The visual phenomena seemed to be exacerbated when he drank coffee.

Dan also noted a lot of unusual three-dimensional effects when looking at colorful flat displays on glossy magazine pages or on his computer screen. Color illustrations started to take on a three-dimensional appearance. One evening, while reading a sailing magazine, he was looking at a photo of an attractive woman wearing a red bikini. The background water was blue. He showed the picture to his wife and asked, "Doesn't it seem like that woman's breasts just pop out of the page, like they're in 3-D?"

Lynn had a look. "Not at all," she said, rolling her eyes.

Over the next several weeks, the visual sensations became more pronounced and more frequent. Dan had no headache or other symptoms. He continued with his research and teaching at Oberlin College, where he was a professor of physics and astronomy. Hoping it might be something like a retinal detachment, he made an appointment to see an optometrist, but everything was normal, including the retinal exam. So, he went to see his internist, Dr. Georgia Newman.

Dr. Newman heard Dan's complaints, examined him, and said, "I'm not sure what's going on. Maybe it's migraine. But it could be a brain tumor. I'm sending you for an MRI."

Her clinical judgment was sharp. Dan had the MRI in a mobile van in a parking lot on Friday afternoon, April 23. When the study was done and Dan was leaving, he asked the radiology technician what the scan showed. She looked stricken. "I'm really not allowed to talk to you," she said. Dan thought that was a bit odd, and it made him feel a little on edge. But aside from the visual flashes, he felt pretty good and left the office having no idea what the MRI showed. He was a little distressed by the look on the radiology technician's face, but he realized there was nothing he could do but wait. So, he decided to put the MRI out of his mind.

In fact, Dan had a very engrossing weekend. A few weeks previously, he and Lynn had bought a sailboat, a used Morgan 28, and Dan was eager to get it back near Oberlin from its current location in LaSalle, Michigan. Not knowing much about boats or sailing, Dan took along Oberlin College physics student Brody Wilson, who did know a few things about boats, to help him make the sixty-mile sail across Lake Erie to Sandusky, Ohio, where they had booked a berth in a marina. As it turned out, the trip across Lake Erie—which can be quite daunting—was easy because there was almost no wind and they motored the whole way, taking twelve hours to complete the journey. At times, Dan thought back to the technician's face when he asked her about the MRI, but the excitement of being on his first boat kept most of those concerns away. Also, being out in the open air and on the water suppressed any visual disturbances he had been having.

Dr. Newman's office called Dan on Tuesday, April 27, and told him he needed to come in for an appointment that afternoon. Dan was concerned and tried to reach Lynn, but she was out of town, teaching at a writers' workshop several hours away. Since they had no cell phones back then, he left a message with a secretary where she was teaching. Once Lynn got the message, she rushed back to accompany him to his 4 p.m. meeting with Dr. Newman.

"Dan, you've got a brain tumor," Dr. Newman said. "And this is the explanation for your symptoms. It's located deep in the brain in the right lateral ventricle, causing a backup of fluid in the ventricle on that side. It will need to be removed. We think it's a rare tumor called a subependymoma."

Dan and Lynn were alarmed and confused. It was the worst-case scenario they could imagine, and it was hard for them to process.

The neuroradiologist who saw the MRI had read an article I had written about minimally invasive approaches to remove certain brain tumors using endoscopes—small telescopes that permit the use of miniaturized instruments. The technique is similar to the way general surgeons use laparoscopes to remove the gallbladder or appendix. She mentioned that article to Dr. Newman, who gave Dan my name and told him to make an appointment to see me.

And that explains how Daniel Stinebring and I met and how he became one of the older patients in my pediatric neurosurgery practice. I proceeded to examine him and found him to be perfectly normal, except for one finding. He had mild papilledema, elevation of the optic discs on ophthalmologic exam, suggestive of increased intracranial pressure.

"Your eyes are okay," I told him. "But there's increased pressure in your head. We need to get that tumor out."

It wasn't completely clear why Dan was seeing stars on his left side, but I thought we had a reasonable explanation. He had normal visual acuity and normal visual fields. The fact that he saw the flashing lights in the left visual field of both eyes suggested that the problem was on the right side of his brain and was retrochiasmatic, behind the optic chiasm (Greek: *khiasmo*, or "a crossing"). That's the site in the brain where the two optic nerves intersect. In front of the optic chiasm, the visual fibers come separately through the optic nerve from each eye before they join. Behind the optic chiasm, the visual fibers are carried in the optic tracts and optic radiations to the primary visual cortex located in the medial occipital lobes at the back of the brain. Hence, the left visual field from each eye is projected to the right occipital cortex, and the right visual field from each eye is projected to the left occipital cortex.

The stars that Dan saw are called photopsias (Greek: *photizein*, "to give light," and *opsia*, "to see"). Photopsias are visual hallucinations that occur when you see flashes of light without light entering the eye. Photopsia itself is a non-specific finding and can be caused by a problem anywhere along the optic pathway from the eye to the visual cortex in the occipital lobe of the brain. The similar term, phosphene (Greek: *phos*, "light," and *phainein*, " to show") describes flashes of light that are more intense and shorter in duration. In general terms, photopsia is the phenomenon of seeing stars, and phosphene describes the individual flashes of light.

The phosphenes that Dan saw were intensely bright, sparkling, unformed, and short-lived. He also saw bright, vibrant colors, sometimes shimmering, sometimes with three-dimensional effects. By carefully logging his symptoms in a journal, Dan was able to localize the problem for us. The fact that the twinkling he saw was retrochiasmatic, behind the optic chiasm, and homonymous, in the same (in this case, left) visual field of both eyes means that the problem was on the right side of the brain.

The MRI showed that Dan's tumor was in the right lateral ventricle, blocking the outflow of cerebrospinal fluid, causing unilateral enlargement of the right lateral ventricle. There were signal changes around the ventricle, confirming that the adjacent brain tissue was under pressure. Behind the optic chiasm, the right optic tract and optic radiations pass near the ventricle as they approach the visual cortex in the occipital lobe. The unilateral enlargement of the right lateral ventricle would explain why Dan's visual hallucinations were noted in the contralateral left visual field. By describing his symptoms in exquisite detail, Dan was telling us where to pinpoint the problem in his brain.

Dan's visual presentation was a little unusual, but it led Dr. Newman to investigate further. She made the wise decision to send him for the MRI. I put the scan up on my lightbox and pointed out the tumor, deep in the right lateral ventricle of the brain. It was obstructing the foramen of Monro, a narrow channel that drains the lateral ventricle into the third ventricle. It was sitting directly on top of the fornix, the memory bundle. And it was causing unilateral obstructive hydrocephalus, a backup of cerebrospinal fluid (CSF) in the right lateral ventricle. The reason for this is that the CSF is a filtrate from blood made by the choroid plexus, a vascular, reddish velvet-like structure in each of the four cerebral ventricles. The human body makes about half a quart of CSF every day. The CSF in Dan's right lateral ventricle wasn't flowing normally because its egress was partially blocked by the tumor. The tumor didn't enhance following the administration of intravenous gadolinium contrast.

I could see the troubled look on their faces as Dan and Lynn saw the deep-seated tumor for the first time. "Don't worry," I said. "We can get this out. But I don't think it's a subependymoma. That's an extremely rare tumor. I want to show this to our neuroradiologists."

So, I brought the films down the hall to Neuroradiology and left Dan and Lynn sitting alone in my office for twenty minutes that I suspect must have felt more like an excruciating hour to them. By now, Dan and Lynn were growing very worried but kept reassuring themselves that the problem could be handled endoscopically. Down the hall, the neuroradiologists and I agreed that the appearance of the tumor was unusual, but we concluded that it had to come out. "We agree it's a tumor," I told Dan and Lynn when I returned. "But we don't think it's a subependymoma. More likely, it's another more common type of tumor, a neurocytoma, astrocytoma, or ependymoma." I realized I was rattling off a bunch of words that were likely meaningless to Dan and Lynn. Those are all primary tumors that arise from the substance of the brain.

"We were sent to you so you could remove it endoscopically, with minimal invasiveness," Lynn said. "Can you do that?"

"Yes, we can do an endoscopic procedure through a small opening in the skull," I said. "But in this case, I wouldn't recommend it. This is a tricky tumor, which sits next to the vascular choroid plexus, which makes the CSF, and abuts the fornix, the bundles of memory. There are risks of bleeding and memory loss. I recommend a small craniotomy. We would do an interhemispheric endoscope-assisted microsurgical resection. We would work in between the two hemispheres of the brain under guidance of the operating microscope and use the endoscope to look around blind corners. I think the small craniotomy would be safer. If any bleeding were to occur, it will be easier for us to stop it. The procedure involves a little larger scalp incision and a little larger bone flap. We'll replace the bone at the end of the procedure. And the hair we have to shave will grow back. The goal is to be minimally invasive to the brain, not so much the bone. We'll get you back to the observatory so the stars you see will be in the sky. We're going to follow the bank robber's credo: get in, get the goods, and get out."

We planned to do the surgery four days later on Friday, May 14, 1999. Lynn expressed surprise that the surgery had to be done so soon. I explained that if the tumor grew just a bit larger, it would close off the egress of the CSF, and that would cause the fluid to accumulate rapidly in the brain, a situation that could be fatal. With that news, suddenly Friday seemed to be a long time away to both Lynn and Dan.

I went over the risks and benefits and answered all their questions. Dan would be admitted to the hospital on Thursday night—that was back in the day when patients could come into the hospital the day before surgery. Lynn would be able to spend the night with him in his room. They shared their anxieties with me, and I did my best to reassure them—we would see Dan through every step of the surgery and recovery. I shared my anxiety with them, noting that I'd have to be extra careful while operating on a high-functioning astrophysicist to dissect the tumor off of his memory fibers. When they left, I gave Dan an article I had written describing the minimally invasive surgical procedure we were about to perform.

That evening, around 10 p.m., I called Dan and Lynn at home to check on them and to see if they had any questions. Lynn answered the phone. When I said, "Hi, this is Big Al (the professional name I go by with my pediatric patients)," she seemed confused. However, once I clarified that I was Dan's neurosurgeon, we had a very nice chat. Lynn told me later that they were surprised that a neurosurgeon would take the time to check on them after their initial appointment. It reminded me of my childhood, watching Ben Casey. I lamented that the surly reputation of neurosurgeons of yesteryear may still linger, though I would like to believe that if Casey were working today, he would likely call his patients too.

Later in the week, Dan told me he had read my article with great enthusiasm, and he emailed me an article he had written about his research specialty, pulsars—ultradense, rotating neutron stars with radio lighthouse beams. The topic was fascinating, but the report was filled with a lot of complex mathematics. I called Dan and confessed that I didn't understand a word of his article and that I would need a translator to explain it to me. But it did serve to remind me how smart he was and how nerve-racking it would be to carry out the surgery. The purpose of the operation was to prevent the potentially devastating consequences if the tumor were to enlarge, block all the ventricles, and cause life-threatening increased intracranial pressure. But Dan's memory was already functioning at the highest level, and there was no way we were going to make it any better. He knew, and we knew, that he had a lot to lose.

Dan had grown up in Pittsburgh, Pennsylvania, where his dad was a microbiologist. He became interested in astronomy when he was a young boy. One day, when he was ten years old, his dad took him out after dark in the backyard of their suburban house on a cul-de-sac. They had a plastic protractor with a string and a metal nut hanging down. His dad showed him how to sight along the protractor at Polaris, the North Star, also known as the Pole Star, since it sits almost directly above the Earth's north pole. The term comes from the Latin, *stella polaris,* for polar star. Polaris marks the end of the handle of Ursa Minor (Little Bear), known as the Little Dipper. It is noteworthy because it appears to hold still while the rest of the northern sky moves around it.

Dan's dad showed him how to pinch the string against the protractor to "take a reading" and then determine their latitude within a degree or so by looking at the protractor dial. That left a lasting impression on Dan. He was hooked. He could use the stars to make meaningful measurements.

It was years later, as an undergraduate student at Williams College, that Dan decided that astronomy would be his future. His astronomy professor, Jay Pasachoff, took him and three other students to view and gather data from a total solar eclipse in far northern Kenya. It was a National Science Foundation-sponsored expedition, and they were the only small college group in the twelve-institution expedition. Dan got to watch the longest total solar eclipse of the last century—over seven minutes of gorgeous, mind-boggling totality. And he was doing it in a remote part of the globe that he had never imagined visiting. Dan turned twenty years old on that expedition and thought, If this is what astronomers do for a living, I'm there!

Dan and Lynn first crossed paths in an unconventional setting. They met while skinny-dipping in the Ithaca Reservoir in the late 1970s. Both were graduate students at Cornell. Lynn liked to joke that when you meet skinny-dipping, you have to get married because it's fun later to shock your teenage children with the story. By 1999, Dan and Lynn's children were not quite teenagers. Anna-Claire was twelve years old, and Jesse was eight. Lynn was a poet and nonfiction writer who would later join the faculty of Oberlin College too.

Dan would go on to earn a master's degree and a PhD at Cornell before joining the faculty at Oberlin College, where he rose to the rank of professor of astrophysics and served as an award-winning teacher and accomplished researcher.

His wife, Lynn, was equally accomplished. Born and raised in Chattanooga, Tennessee, she earned her BA at Carson Newman College in Jefferson City, Tennessee, and an MFA at Cornell, where she met her future husband. Her years at Cornell marked the first time she had been north of the Mason-Dixon line.

We scheduled Dan's surgery to be carried out in my OR in the Children's Hospital on Friday, May 14, 1999. He would be admitted to the adjacent adult hospital, where he would also recover. I went to visit Dan in his room at 10:30 p.m. the night before his surgery to answer any questions. I was accompanied by Shekar Kurpad, my senior resident at the time, who would assist me in the OR the next day. Shekar was a superb resident who had earned his MD and PhD from Duke. I introduced him to Lynn and Dan using his nickname, *Shaky*, which I had given him years earlier as a term of endearment. When I heard myself saying it out loud, I realized that it was not the wisest choice of a nickname for a neurosurgeon, and I had to clarify to the family that it had nothing to do with his operative skills.

A portable cot had been delivered to the room for Lynn to sleep on, but it was stuck in a folded position, and she was having trouble opening it. So, I bent over and started to undo the latch. She quickly pushed me away, saying, "I think the cot is booby-trapped. Please don't touch it. We can't let anything bad to happen to your hands." We all had a good laugh. Shaky and I answered more of their questions, and we left to prepare for the next morning.

Lynn was clearly nervous. She'd only had a few days to process the brain surgery her husband was about to undergo, and she was aware of the risks. Her mind was racing, and she thought about the possibility of becoming a widow in her forties and of Anna-Claire and Jesse losing their father. Lynn's parents had driven the five hundred miles from Tennessee to babysit. Because in talking to their kids, Dan and Lynn had focused not on the risks of surgery but on the surgery making their dad feel better, the kids were handling the situation reasonably well. Jesse was excited that their dad had gotten his head shaved for the surgery. The family had been planning a trip to South Carolina the next month, and he thought it was funny that his dad would be bald on Bald Head Island.

On the morning of surgery, Lynn felt apprehensive but grateful when the attentive nurses came to pick up Dan and take him to the OR. He had to be wheeled over to the Children's Hospital on a stretcher, through the basement. Dan had received no sedation that morning, but he was his usual laid-back self, chatting away constantly with the nurses. Lynn left him in the basement. She had no idea what to expect but got some sense of relief watching her husband go calmly and happily down the corridor, talking nonstop.

In the OR, Dan continued chatting with the anesthesiologists, who explained what was going to happen to him over the next six hours. He was a little taken aback but smiled as he looked up and saw dinosaurs lining the walls of the operating theater. I prefer to do my surgical procedures in the Children's OR, even when my patient is an adult. I'm more comfortable there because I work with the same team, day in and day out.

In the OR, the neurosurgeon is the captain of the ship. He sets the tone for the room and must ensure that everyone is rowing in the same direction. I like to play music because it creates a relaxed atmosphere, and I think everyone functions better when they are relaxed. I tailor the playlist for the specific operative case, but some things remain constant. During induction of anesthesia, we often play "Stayin' Alive" by the Bee Gees. We usually start the case with "Smooth Operator" by Sade. And if we time things right, James Brown's "I Feel Good" comes on once the tumor has been removed.

Some surgeons prefer to operate in complete silence and feel it improves their ability to concentrate on every minute detail of the procedure. I don't begrudge them for that. But I prefer to choreograph my surgeries, and I feel music helps everyone in the room relax and work more effectively together as a team. That said, in every case, the overarching goal of the entire OR staff is to get the patient safely and swiftly through the surgery and out of the room.

The optimal surgical case is carefully orchestrated. The surgical planning is carried out before the patient enters the room, and the procedure is rehearsed during a time-out at the beginning of each case. The surgeon is always thinking several steps in advance to make the case go smoothly and to prepare for potential pitfalls that might occur. When things are going well, I can keep my eyes on the operative field, hold up my hand, and the scrub nurse will give me the instrument I need without me even having to ask for it. The best surgeon isn't necessarily the one who operates the fastest. The best surgeon learns to use economy of movement so that one segment of the procedure appears to blend effortlessly into the next without intervening downtime.

We carried out Dan's surgery through a right frontal craniotomy and interhemispheric transcallosal approach to the tumor.[1] This enabled us to get down to the tumor deep in the center of Dan's head without having to disrupt the cerebral cortex or deep white matter. We could work through a small opening in the corpus callosum under high magnification. The tumor was in the lateral ventricle, just above the thalamus.

The challenge presented by Dan's tumor was twofold. First, it blocked the foramen of Monro, the passage from the lateral ventricle to the third ventricle, like a ball blocking the drain of a sink. This created hydrocephalus, a backup of fluid in the lateral ventricle, which increased the intracranial pressure and affected his visual fibers, causing Dan to see stars in the daytime. Second, and just as serious, it was adherent to the fornix (Latin for "arch"), the bundle of fibers that carries memory from the hippocampus to the hypothalamus. The hippocampus (Greek:

---

1 This was the same corridor we used to remove Emma's thalamic brain tumor in Chapter 3.

hippos, "horse," and *kampos*, "sea monster") is embedded deep in the temporal lobe and has the shape of a sea horse. Its major function is concerned with learning and memory. So, our job was to peel the tumor off the memory bundle of an astrophysicist who had a perfectly functioning memory going into surgery. The entire surgical team was on edge, especially me.

The surgical technique we used in Dan's case was endoscope-assisted microsurgery. Using the operating microscope on high power, we made a small opening in the anterior corpus callosum—the white matter tract that connects the two hemispheres of the brain—and entered the right lateral ventricle. This gave us an excellent view of the grayish, glassy, moderately vascular tumor sitting on the fornix and obstructing the outflow of the ventricle downstream into the foramen of Monro. By using the endoscope, a thin surgical telescope with angled lenses, we could look around the back of the tumor as we removed it from the adjacent crucial brain structures.

The surgery went smoothly, and we were able to sneak in and get the tumor out without any obvious visible injury to the memory bundle. The frozen section biopsy came back to us while we were still in the OR as subependymoma. This was the exact diagnosis predicted by the neuroradiologist at Oberlin, the same diagnosis that our neuroradiology team had dismissed, because it is statistically so uncommon. The overall incidence of subependymoma is about one-half of 1 percent of tumors of the nervous system. Damn, I thought, Oberlin was right. We were wrong.

Subependymoma is a very rare benign WHO grade 1 tumor that can be found in the ventricles, often in middle-aged or older patients, usually in men. It arises from the ependyma (Greek for "upper garment"), a single layer of ciliated columnar epithelial cells that form the lining of the ventricles.

Lynn had brought two friends to stay with her in the waiting room, but her anxiety level was very high, and time seemed to go painfully slowly. After several long hours, she got a call from a nurse in the OR, letting her know that things were going well. At the end of the case, I came out and brought Lynn to Dan's bedside in the Neurosurgery Intensive Care Unit. He was lying on his back with his eyes closed. The white turban we had placed on his head made him look dignified. I rubbed his chest gently, and he opened his eyes immediately. "Hi, Big Al," he said with a broad smile. "So good to see you!" Dan turned to Lynn, who tearfully squeezed his hand. Lynn and I smiled, relieved to know that his brain was working fine.

"Good news," I said. "We got the tumor out. It's a subependymoma. WHO grade 1. Benign!"

"Way to go Oberlin!" Dan belted out, reminding everyone within earshot that my team of experts had guessed incorrectly about the diagnosis, while his team was spot on. A week later, the permanent pathology report would come back, after all the special stains had been done, confirming the diagnosis of subependymoma.

We went on to do a post-op exam in the ICU, and it was clear that all circuits were firing correctly. He was speaking fluently and lucidly, his cranial nerves were intact, and he moved all extremities well. But what about his memory? We usually test this by asking patients some basic questions about current events or having them perform some simple arithmetic exercises in addition or subtraction. But that wouldn't work here.

Dan was no ordinary patient. He was an astrophysicist, and we had just peeled a brain tumor off his memory bundles. How could we assess the nuances of memory in someone who could do simple mathematical calculations in his sleep? We needed to improvise. Fortunately, we had anticipated this problem and had come prepared with a plan.

When he awakened from surgery, we planned to ask Dan to recite the Fibonacci sequence. If he could do that, we knew his memory was all there. This sequence, attributed to the thirteenth-century mathematician Leonardo Fibonacci of Pisa, is a series of steadily increasing numbers beginning with zero, in which each number is the sum of the preceding two numbers. It is a powerful sequence in mathematics from which the Golden Ratio is derived.

The Golden Ratio is the ratio of a given number in the sequence divided by its predecessor. It approximates the number 1.618, written as the Greek letter phi. The Golden Ratio is considered to be the most aesthetically perfect and pleasing proportion in nature and art. Some refer to it as Nature's Code. It is considered to represent the harmony of the universe, explaining why it has also been called the Divine Proportion. The Golden Ratio can be seen all around us, in the branching of trees, the number of petals on a flower, the shell of a snail, the spiral arms of a galaxy, the spin of a hurricane, the pyramids of Giza, and even the face of the Mona Lisa.

"The Fibonacci sequence? Guys, that's the best you can come up with?" Dan asked, rattling off the series perfectly: "0, 1, 1, 2, 3, 5, 8, 13, 21, 34, 55..." with the panache of an entertainer who was clearly showing off and enjoying himself, until we cut him off. We were impressed. And we were relieved. Who knows how long he could have gone on?

Lynn spent two hours in the ICU, watching Dan's monitors religiously as he slept. Reassured that he was okay, Lynn left to spend the night with friends in town. She called to check on him the next morning at about 4 a.m. He was already wide awake and full of energy, euphoric on steroids, writing letters to friends, and reading a book. She came in to visit him at 9 a.m. but was unnerved when she found his ICU bed empty.

"Is he getting an MRI?" she asked. "No," the nurse told her. "He had the MRI last night, and it showed the tumor was gone." He's walked out of the ICU. We've lost control of him. Lynn was apprehensive because the staff had no idea where he was. Could something terrible have happened to him? Could he have wandered off somewhere, gotten into an elevator, left the floor, and gotten lost? After a few fretful minutes, she was relieved to find him out walking the floors in his hospital gown, pushing his IV pole, peeved that the ICU nurses didn't have enough time to talk to him. He was chitchatting with a group of strangers in the hallway. He was high on life, amped up on perioperative steroids, telling Lynn he felt as if he had superpowers.

Gradually, Dan started to come down a bit from his blissful state of mania as his postoperative steroids were tapered. He was discharged home after three days. It took a while for his energy to come back, and he had some difficulty with his wake-sleep cycle, but he was well enough to fly to a conference of the American Astronomical Society with his students in Chicago ten days after his surgery.

Dan was energized at the meeting, still pumped up from having come through the surgery okay. He had T-shirts made that he and his students wore showing pictures of his MRI before and after the tumor resection. He proudly showed off his bald head and craniotomy scar. But while his intellect was spot on, his judgment took a little more time to come back. The first night in his Chicago hotel, while he was alone in his room, he had trouble sleeping, so he took an Ambien along with a warm bath and started drifting off to sleep. Fortunately, he woke up abruptly and quickly got himself out of the tub, avoiding disaster, but not a stern scolding from Lynn when he reported to her his mistake.

When Dan got back from the meeting in Chicago, he was still invigorated and decided to go outside and mow the lawn. Unfortunately, he managed to smack his head on a low-lying branch, which gave both Dan and Lynn headaches. Dan had a mild concussion but was able to bounce back quickly.

Dan resumed his work at Oberlin, where he was very popular among the faculty and students. He received stacks of get-well cards from friends and family, many of whom shared his unique sense of humor. John, one of his colleagues, wrote him the following email message:

> By the way Dan, I understand that this tumor may have had a slight effect on your short-term memory. In case you have forgotten, I wanted to remind you that the week before you went in for surgery you told me that you lost your sailboat to me in a bet. Shall I stop over and pick up the keys or do you want to drop them off?

Fortunately for Dan, his memory was working fine, and he was able to hold on to the boat he had never sold in the first place.

One month after surgery, Dan took Lynn and their kids on vacation, as promised, to Bald Head Island in South Carolina. He was the only one who was appropriately coiffed, and he was able to show off his scar while his hair was starting to grow back.

Three months after surgery, Dan came for a follow-up MRI and exam. Everything was fine, and I showed him the scan and assured him the tumor was gone. The next day, he sent me the following email:

> I had a bit of an adventure after I left your office yesterday. I went to your medical center's athletic facility to give Lynn a call. I asked the attendant for directions to a pay phone (Author's note: This was a quarter century ago, before the widespread use of cell phones). He told me it was in the locker room, and I went in and found it. Part way through placing my call I looked over and saw a woman, scantily clad, brushing her hair in front of a mirror. Oops, wrong locker room! Fortunately, I got out of there before anyone screamed, although three women who were coming into the locker room as I left (in front of the big sign that said WOMEN) gave me a bit of a grilling about why I was in there. Maybe the brain surgery wasn't so successful after all.

Four months after surgery, Dan gave me a book called *The Divine Proportion: A Study in Mathematical Beauty*, by H.E. Huntley, a professor from Somerset, UK. The book begins with a striking radiograph of the shell of the chambered nautilus *(Nautilus pompillius)*, a marine mollusk found in the Indo-Pacific Ocean. The nautilus (from the Ancient Greek *nautilos*, "sailor") uses jet propulsion to roam the floor of the sea. The nautilus shell has a framework of successive chambers based on a logarithmic spiral. The animal lives in the largest shell chamber, and the smaller chambers act like the ballast tanks of a submarine to propel the nautilus. The nautilus shell is a reminder of the grace of nature—the Divine Proportion. As the shell grows, the size of the chambers increases, but their shape remains unaltered. The relationship between successive chambers is an example of the Golden Ratio, based on the Fibonacci sequence we used to assess the function of Dan Stinebring's memory after his brain tumor resection.

Six months after surgery, I gave grand rounds in Severance Hall at Oberlin College. Dan and his colleague, Mark Braford, a professor of biology and neuroscience, had invited me to speak about minimally invasive neurosurgery. With Dan's permission, I showed photographs and videos of his brain tumor resection. Dan spoke as well. I can't imagine what it must have been like to talk to a large group about your own brain surgery. If one considers the term introspection as the examination of one's own mental processes, then that day, Dan Stinebring must have had the ultimate experience in introspection. How many of us have had the opportunity to watch a video of our own memory fibers pulsating away on a large screen in front of an audience and then describe what the process was like? That is a true out-of-body experience.

We each spoke about the common threads of our two professions. I was struck by the fact that the magnetic resonance image (MRI) scanner we used to diagnose Dan's brain tumor was a tool developed by physicists and one of the topics Dan lectured on in some of his advanced physics classes. It was a fun day and one of the most unusual sessions I have ever been part of.

Dan and his family have remained in touch with me over the years. I followed him annually with surveillance MRIs for a time that showed no evidence of recurrent tumor. His memory has been perfect. He has traveled around the world, working with various radio telescopes to study the stars of the cosmos.

He sent me one of his articles about orthogonal modes of polarization in pulsar radio emission, thanking me for keeping him in the game. It was a kind gesture, but I still didn't understand a word he wrote.

Dan and I have remained close. Our careers have followed an interesting parallel. He was awarded an endowed chair at Oberlin, the Francis D. Federighi Professorship in Physics and Astronomy, and he invited me to the ceremony. Soon after, I was awarded an endowed chair at my medical center, and he and Lynn came to celebrate with me.

Like her husband, Lynn went on to join the faculty at Oberlin, where she served as the founding director of Writers in the Schools (WITS), which trains students to teach creative writing in schools. Over the years, she has taught a wide range of poetry and nonfiction courses at the college and has authored three award-winning books of poetry. She also authored a nonfiction book, *Framing Innocence: A Mother's Photographs, a Prosecutor's Zeal, and a Small Town's Response,* which won the Studs and Ida Terkel Award from the New Press. This was a powerful story detailing how a caring community stood up against an unjust prosecution. Among her numerous awards was a Literature Fellowship for the National Endowment for the Arts.

Dan and Lynn have been happily married for over forty years. They have spent a good deal of time sailing on their boat, *Polaris*, going up to the North Channel of Lake Huron, enjoying the serene north country. Their son Jesse, who was eight years old at the time of Dan's surgery, is now thirty-five. He is a founder and the CEO of Blue Rose Research, a cutting-edge data analytics firm serving the Democratic and progressive world. He has completed two Ironman races with his family cheering him on. Jesse's wife, Zaib, whom he married in 2023, works for the United States Treasury Department on counter-illicit finance policy.

Dan and Lynn's daughter, Anna-Claire, who was twelve at the time of her dad's surgery, is now thirty-nine She earned her PhD in the history of art at the University of Pennsylvania and is now a curator of European paintings at the Metropolitan Museum of Art. Her husband, Adam, is a psychiatric mental health nurse practitioner.

Dan is still actively in the game as a stargazer. Since his surgery, he no longer sees those stars in the daytime, except when he works with his radio telescopes. Unlike optical telescopes, which analyze visible light waves, radio telescopes analyze cosmic waves with frequencies in a different part of the electromagnetic spectrum and can also be used in the daytime. But the floating stars he used to see in the shower are forever gone.

Dan has continued to do groundbreaking work in astrophysics. He is a senior member of the North American Nanohertz Observatory for Gravitational Waves (NANOGrav), focused on studying low-frequency gravitational waves. They are concentrating on the detection of low-frequency gravitational waves, elusive ripples in the framework of space and time that are produced by thousands of orbiting pairs of supermassive black holes.

These supermassive black holes, some of which are millions to billions of times more massive than our sun, sit at the core of galaxies. Galaxies (Greek: *gala*, "milk"), like our own spiral Milky Way, are giant clusters of billions of stars, planets, and interstellar gas and dust bound together by gravity. Galaxies grow when they become close to one another and eventually merge. When this happens, the supermassive black holes at their core become paired and begin to spin around each other, emitting giant rippling waves at the speed of light over the pond of spacetime.

The vibration of gravitational waves in the fabric of spacetime is analogous to the formation of sound waves from the vibration of air molecules.

In July 2023, Dan and over one hundred collaborators at NANOGrav from around the world reported the finding of a low-pitched cosmic symphony of gigantic gravitational waves emanating from thousands of pairs of supermassive black holes. This discovery has laid to rest any prior perception of a static universe. The finding is based on data painstakingly collected over fifteen years from multiple radio telescopes around the world.

The information was gleaned by studying dozens of pulsars up to twenty thousand light-years away. By analyzing tiny deviations in the radio waves emitted from these ultra-accurate celestial pulsar "time clocks," NANOGrav scientists were able to demonstrate the presence of the faint ripples of spacetime, the so-called gravitational waves. Their discovery lends support to Albert Einstein's general theory of relativity, which he formulated over a century ago, in 1916, predicting the presence of gravitational waves rippling the fabric of the universe.

The tight-knit, remarkably collegial NANOGrav collaborators published their results in the *Astrophysical Journal*, hoping that their analysis of these gravitational waves would provide insights about the history of the cosmos. The novel findings should help shed light on the early inflationary expansion of the universe following the giant fireball of the Big Bang 13.7 billion years ago. It will also tell us more about the formation of our giant galaxies.

As a stargazer, Dan is also a time-traveler. The gravitational waves he studies originated in the far distant past. Carl Sagan reminds us, "The immense distances to the stars and the galaxies mean that we see everything in space in the past—some as they were before the Earth came to be. Telescopes are time machines."

With his time machine, Dan Stinebring continues to look back in the past to tell us more about the present and the future. A quarter century after his brain surgery, Dan avidly pursues his journey, listening to gravitational whispers in order to unravel some of the deepest mysteries of the universe. He is a brilliant man from whom I have learned many valuable lessons about courage, kindness, and humility.

CHAPTER 7

Humor

"As soap is to the body, so laughter is to the soul."

JEWISH PROVERB

It was a cold, blustery morning as I was driving to work at Johns Hopkins Hospital on Thursday, January 19, 2017, and I was looking forward to a quiet day. It had been a busy week. I had operated on three children with brain tumors over the past two days and had been in the OR from dawn till dusk each day. One child was a fourteen-year-old girl with headaches from a large chondroma, a benign cartilaginous skull tumor compressing the right frontal lobe. One was a sixteen-year-old girl with seizures from a dysembryoplastic neuroepithelial tumor (DNET), a benign tumor that involves the cerebral cortex and white matter of the brain. And the third was a sixteen-year-old boy with a large disfiguring left frontotemporal skull mass that proved to be fibrous dysplasia, a disorder in which the bone is replaced by scar-like connective tissue.

All three of them were doing well, and the rest of our inpatient service was stable. I was planning to spend the day seeing patients in the clinic and catching up on office work.

Listening to the radio on the way in, I was captivated by the lead news story of the day. Joaquin Guzman, better known to the world as "El Chapo" (Shorty), the infamous Mexican drug lord and leader of the Sinaloa Cartel, had been recaptured after his second prison escape and was being extradited to the United States later in the day. I was thinking about what a crazy world we're living in. His escape was something out of a Hollywood thriller movie.

On February 22, 2014, the date of his recapture following an extensive manhunt, he was remanded to a solitary windowless room in the Mexican Altiplano Federal Maximum Security Prison. He was able to break out through a small hole in the floor of his cell by his shower, the only site in the room that was in the blind spot of the twenty-four-hour surveillance provided by the security camera in his room. He climbed down a ladder into a mile-long lighted tunnel with air ducts created by his co-conspirators, using a motorcycle to transport himself through the tunnel to safety. Now, following his recapture and extradition to the US, the plan was to house him for the rest of his life in a "Supermax" prison from which no one had ever escaped.

It was an incredible, mind-boggling story. But as crazy as it was, that day I was laser-focused on the upcoming weekend. In two days, I was scheduled to leave for the annual meeting of the American Society of Pediatric Neurosurgeons (ASPN). The ASPN is one of my favorite organizations. Each year, in the middle of winter, a group of senior pediatric neurosurgeons from across the country gets together to showcase their research and discuss the state-of-the-art of our field.

The talks are in the mornings and are no-holds-barred, meaning that the presenters can be roundly critiqued by the senior listeners in attendance. The time allocated for discussion is always longer than that allocated for the talk. After a congenial but sometimes raucous and bruising morning, the members can then spend time with their friends and families in the afternoons and evenings. I was slated to give an invited talk, which I hadn't yet prepared. I was planning to put the talk together in the time remaining before I flew out.

One thing that's certain in the life of a pediatric neurosurgeon is that nothing is ever certain. The day started off normally, without any surprises. I attended several conferences in the hospital, made rounds on my patients, and spent the rest of the day in my outpatient clinic. Later in the afternoon, I got a phone call from an endocrinologist, Dr. Debra Counts, from one of our neighboring hospitals, asking if I could have a look at a young boy that she was sending over to our hospital with a newly diagnosed giant brain tumor.

And that's how I came to meet Declan Ambrose in our emergency room. He was a delightful, spunky five-year-old boy who would come to change my life as much as I changed his. He was clearly apprehensive and had no interest in being in the hospital's emergency room. His pediatrician, Dr. Jeffries Bucci, had observed that Declan had exceptionally short stature for his age. Declan had also been having progressively more severe bifrontal headaches and fatigue over the past eight months. Dr. Bucci referred him to Dr. Counts, who sent off some blood work and found that Declan's growth hormone level was low.

Looking for the cause of his short stature, Dr. Counts sent him for a cranial MRI. The MRI was done earlier in the day and showed a very large midline mass at the base of Declan's brain. Dr. Counts called the family and told them, "We saw something on the scan we didn't like that needs further evaluation." Then she called me and sent Declan over to our ER for an urgent visit.

Aside from short stature and some anxiety, Declan looked to me like a normal five-year-old boy. The ophthalmology team examined him and noted a mild bilateral superior temporal quadrantic visual field cut. This was likely caused by the large mass pressing on his optic chiasm, where the eye fibers from the right and left visual fields cross in the center of the brain. By compressing the crossing fibers in the optic chiasm, the tumor had created a modified form of tunnel vision, knocking out the upper outer fields of vision on each side.

After examining Declan, I sat down with his parents, Stevi and Brian, reviewed the history, and went over the MRI with them. The phone call from Dr. Counts that afternoon had turned their lives upside down. They were a happy, easygoing family and had never before had to deal with any significant health-related issues. They had two healthy boys, Declan and his younger brother Oliver. Stevi and Brian had good, stable jobs that were equally unusual. Stevi worked at the American Visionary Art Museum in Baltimore, described by CNN as "one of the most fantastic museums anywhere in America." The museum featured unique exhibitions that combined art, science, philosophy, social justice, and humor. Brian worked in the marketing department for Zeni Max Media, a large-scale video games manufacturer. This was the first real crisis either of them had ever faced.

It was obvious from the scan that Declan had a giant brain tumor. It was a complex, cystic and solid, lobulated, contrast-enhancing, expansile mass situated in the midline at the base of Declan's skull. It had obstructed the cerebral ventricles to cause severe hydrocephalus with increased intracranial pressure. It compressed the optic chiasm and spilled out under both frontal lobes, pushing them upward and compressing them. It also spilled out laterally into the left middle cranial fossa, putting pressure on the temporal lobe. The tumor had calcifications around its periphery with heavy calcification centrally, confirmed via a CT scan we obtained later that evening.

I could see the fear in Stevi and Brian's eyes as they stared in disbelief at the images of their young son's brain. "How could something this big be inside his head?" Stevi asked. "How can he be walking and talking with a scan looking like this?" It was a good question, I thought. I had been wondering the same thing.

Stevi started to blame herself. "How could I have not picked this up earlier? Declan was always short. I thought it ran in our family. His great-grandfather was a talented horse jockey and was really short. And we have other family members who were short. I thought Declan just had the *jockey gene*. I feel I should have done something earlier. I feel I let my son down."

I assured her that was not the case. Slow-growing midline tumors in children can be elusive to diagnose. They can often grow to a very large size before they are detected because they tend to expand underneath the brain in the subarachnoid space, displacing fluid until they become large enough to compress the brain and obstruct drainage from the cerebral ventricles. Also, most headaches in kids are not caused by brain tumors. And visual changes in the young can be difficult to detect, because they come on slowly, and the child may not be aware of them. These are kids who sometimes get moved to the front of the classroom because they have difficulty seeing what's on the blackboard, while the elusive tumor continues its slow, relentless growth.

"I think it's a craniopharyngioma," I said. "That's a benign tumor, but it's in a malignant, dangerous place, right smack in the middle of his brain. These tend to be slow-growing tumors, but Declan's tumor has become so large that it's also blocking his cerebrospinal fluid pathways, causing hydrocephalus. Declan will need surgery so we can be certain of the diagnosis, remove as much of the tumor as is safely possible, and treat his hydrocephalus to relieve the increased pressure it's causing inside his head."

As Stevi and Brian were struggling to make sense of what was happening, Declan's illness also presented an unexpected logistical challenge for me. It put a significant dent in my plans, as I knew I would spend most of the next day in the OR and not be able to prepare my talk. It was Thursday night, and I was leaving town for a meeting on Saturday morning. We talked about the possibility of delaying the operation until I returned, but there was too much risk of something bad happening during the time I would be gone. So, we decided to operate the next morning. We discussed plans with Declan, telling him that we needed to do a procedure to take the pressure off his brain and make him feel better. He was uneasy and not happy about what was happening. He nodded but didn't really understand everything I was saying.

Whenever possible, I try to include the child in the plans for surgery. I think it's important, but there's no one-size-fits all in this approach. It's helpful to gauge how much the child wants to know. And the age of the child certainly matters. I usually begin with a broad comment about the surgery and see how the child responds. Some kids ask a lot of questions, others are stone-cold silent. Either way, I think it's important to have them participate in some fashion, even without going into explicit detail about the potential risks of surgery. Some parents, in an attempt to protect their child, ask me not to mention anything about the surgery. In most cases, I recommend against this tactic. It can increase the child's anxiety and contribute to a loss of the child's trust. Imagine the panic a young patient might experience being wheeled off into a strange OR without knowing why.

Early the next morning, on January 20, 2017, I was driving to work listening again to the news on the radio. This time, it was all about Donald Trump. Later that day, he would be inaugurated as the forty-fifth president of the United States, with arguments to follow about the size of the crowd attending the event. The following day would see an international Women's March in protest of the inauguration, with almost five million participants worldwide. But as was often the case when I was about to start a big operation, I had pretty much zoned out the rest of the world and was focusing on how our team was planning to go after Declan's tumor.

I met Declan in the OR. In spite of all our preparation Declan was scared and crying inconsolably. Stevi had put on a sterile jumpsuit to accompany him to the OR and was standing by his side when the anesthesiologist gently placed a mask on his face to give him a little knockout gas. That didn't go well. Stevi tried to comfort him, but to no avail. He was thrashing around and struggling to sit up and get off the OR table. Things were spiraling out of control.

Then, through a stroke of good fortune, my friend and colleague Ed McKay saw what was going on and sidled up to the OR table. Ed put his hand gently on Declan and, in a calm, soothing voice, asked him if he wanted to look at a *Simpsons* cartoon video. Then Ed, keeping one hand on Declan, pulled out his iPhone and turned on the cartoon. And something magical happened. Declan calmed down immediately and began watching the video. In fact, he became so engrossed in it that he didn't even look up to see his tearful mother leaving the OR as the anesthesia team gently put him under. In that simple act, Ed reminded me of the power of human kindness.

What Ed accomplished in a couple of minutes in the OR demonstrates the importance of compassion and teamwork. Ed isn't a neurosurgeon. He isn't a physician. But he is a remarkable young man. He works as a senior surgical technologist, scrubbing with us in the OR to help make the cases go smoothly. And whenever I see Ed in the room, I breathe a sigh of relief because I know things will go well.

Ed grew up in a tough neighborhood in the city. By the time he graduated from high school, most of his friends had already dropped out. In fact, most had dropped out by the ninth grade. Ed was the guy who made it out of the neighborhood. He got where he is today with a mixture of courage and perseverance. The kids and families in the hospital love him. He actually makes rounds on our patients later in the day when we come out of the OR, and he comes to see them with us when they return to the clinic for follow-up visits.

Ed has also taken the time to give back to those less fortunate than he was, the friends he left behind. He shares his remarkable story with students ranging from elementary school to college. He became inspired while watching a television documentary entitled, *My Brother's Keeper*, and went on to become a mentor with City of Baltimore Children of Incarcerated Parents Program.

Seeing Ed work his magic in the OR that morning was no surprise. That's what he would do as a matter of routine. I was focused more on watching Declan's tearful mother walk out of the OR, leaving her treasured child in our hands. She had met me less than twelve hours earlier, and now she was handing her son over to our team open his head and work deep inside his brain. Things had moved so quickly that she and Brian never had enough time to really understand what was going on. Stevi told me later that when she left the OR that morning, she wasn't sure she would ever see her child again. She believed his tumor was a ticking time bomb.

Her words continue to haunt me. It's hard to imagine how terrifying something like this must be for a parent. But I suspect I've become somewhat numbed because I see it happen so often when we separate the parent and child, either in OR on the way to the OR. I began to experience significant feelings of guilt. On the previous day, I was fixated on my own schedule, trying to put my talk together and prepare for my meeting. What must this poor family have been going through? Why wasn't I more sensitive to their needs? I was embarrassed to have to remind myself to focus more on the patient and family and less on myself.

Pediatric neurosurgery is a very personal field. When things go well, the rewards are always off the scale. When they go badly, it's gut-wrenching. Either way, it's essentially impossible to detach yourself from the circumstances. In many cases, the pediatric neurosurgeon essentially becomes a member of the family, sharing the good times and the bad times. Treating a brain tumor is something that can be done in a methodical fashion, with meticulous, calculated precision. But healing the child and family requires a very different and uniquely personal approach.

I had met with our team early that morning to plan how we would approach Declan's tumor. Because he had significant hydrocephalus, if we were to open the skull in a standard fashion, the brain would be under so much pressure it would herniate out of the head. We decided to do a two-stage synchronous ventriculoscopic and microsurgical resection of the large tumor under the same general anesthesia. It's a technique that we and others had described previously to simplify the removal of complex deep midline cystic and solid brain tumors.

Our aim was to begin with a minimally invasive endoscopic technique to enter the cerebral ventricle from above using a small burr hole exposure in the skull, drain CSF, then open the tumor cyst endoscopically under direct vision to decompress it, take biopsies, and remove some of the upper portion of the tumor. This would reduce the intracranial pressure significantly, enabling us to perform the second stage immediately to follow, a craniotomy at the base of the skull to debulk the tumor working underneath the brain with guidance of the operating microscope.

So, with Declan anesthetized and lying supine, we made a small burr hole in his right frontal skull and introduced a small endoscope into the right lateral ventricle under direct vision and drained CSF. Then we found the tumor, and using microinstruments, we fenestrated the wall of the cystic portion, then taking biopsies of the tumor and making a generous hole in the cyst capsule to decompress the tumor fluid. We left a drainage catheter in the tumor cyst and brought it out of Declan's head to let the fluid accumulate in a sterile bag. This effectively relaxed the brain.

Next, we turned Declan's head to the left and performed a right frontotemporal craniotomy, removing a trap-door piece of his skull that enabled us to gently elevate the brain and debulk the large tumor working through a narrow corridor using the microscope. Parts of the tumor were thick and heavily calcified, stuck to some important real estate, including the optic nerves, carotid arteries, pituitary stalk, and hypothalamus. We were able to get a good resection of the tumor, intentionally leaving some small scraps that were tightly stuck to the vital structures to avoid injuring them. I was working with two senior neurosurgeons, Lee Titsworth and Christina Jackson, and we were all pleased with how things went. It was a long day. The operation lasted nine hours.

While we were closing the head, the frozen section from pathology returned *adamantinomatous craniopharyngioma*. The diagnosis was not a surprise to us. That's exactly what the tumor looked like on the pre-op CT and MRI. And that's what it looked like to us in the OR. The neurosurgeon can never really be 100 percent sure of the diagnosis until the neuropathologists examine the specimen sent to them from the OR. But this tumor had such characteristic features that it couldn't have been anything else.

I spoke to Stevi and Brian in the waiting room and shared the good news—it was a benign tumor, the surgery went well, and Declan was extubated and waking up in the pediatric ICU. Stevi cried. She and Brian were still very worried. They didn't know what to think. They never knew anyone who had undergone brain surgery. They wondered if Declan would be the same child they brought to the hospital the day before.

I took them over to the bedside in the PICU. They saw their son sitting upright with a white turban on his head, complaining that he was thirsty. He was feisty and said he wanted real water, not the "stupid wet sponge on a stick" that the nurse had given him to suck on. That was the time, Stevi told me later, that she knew the old Declan was back and that he was going to be okay.

Although the craniopharyngioma is a benign tumor, it is, in my opinion, the most difficult tumor we deal with in pediatric neurosurgery because of its central location in the head. Craniopharyngiomas are rare neoplasms, accounting for about 2 percent of all childhood brain tumors. They tend to arise near the stalk of the pituitary gland and can cause a variety of symptoms, including headache, vomiting, and visual and endocrine disturbances.

The first reported case of a craniopharyngioma was by the German pathologist Friedrich Albert von Zenker in 1857. He described it in an autopsy as a "cystic suprasellar mass containing cholesterol crystals and squamous epithelium." The term craniopharyngioma was coined by Harvey Cushing in 1929, who later described it as "the most forbidding of the intracranial tumors." The word is a portmanteau, an amalgamation of cranio (Greek: *kranion*, "skull") and pharyngioma (Greek: *pharynx*, "throat").

Craniopharyngiomas are considered low-grade tumors, WHO grade 1, and have a bimodal distribution, affecting children in the first decade of life and adults in their fifth decade. There are two histologic types of craniopharyngioma: adamantinomatous and papillary. Adamantinomatous craniopharyngiomas primarily affect children, while the papillary variant more is more commonly seen in adults. More recently, craniopharyngiomas, like other brain tumors, are being characterized on a molecular level in the hope of finding targetable mutations to improve treatment. Adamantinomatous craniopharyngiomas may have mutations in exon 3 of *CTNNB1*, the gene encoding the protein β-catenin which activates a WNT tumor signaling pathway. Papillary craniopharyngiomas may have mutations in the *BRAF* V600E oncogene (a mutated gene that can drive formation of tumors). The alphabet soup of molecular biology is changing the landscape of brain tumor categorization and management.

The term adamantinomatous comes from the word adamant (Latin: *adamas*, "hard steel"), emphasizing the firm nature of these tumors, which are partially calcified and can be adherent to the critical neurovascular brain structures that surround them at the skull base. This is what makes their removal treacherous and their recurrence rate high. The reason the adamantinomatous variant of craniopharyngioma is so firm is that its calcification arises from ameloblasts, a group of epithelial cells that normally produce the enamel that forms on developing teeth.

Declan's post-op course was smooth. His headaches resolved, and he had no visual complaints or weakness. He got a nice visit from Mozart, the golden retriever pet therapy dog, who sat on the bed with Declan and watched *Scooby-Doo* on TV with him. Declan also got a visit from Ed McKay when he woke up from surgery. Ed brought him a Spiderman coloring book and some crayons and continued to visit him every day during his lunch break.

Declan's post-op MRI looked good, with significant decompression of the bulk of the tumor, which took the pressure off his brain. He did develop excessive thirst and urination (diabetes insipidus, or water diabetes), which we controlled by giving him vasopressin, a pituitary hormone that prevents water loss by the kidneys, and he required hydrocortisone and thyroid replacement. Such hormone replacement is common after surgical resection of craniopharyngiomas and other tumors adjacent to the hypothalamus, the master gland. But Declan bounced back quickly and was out of intensive care in a few days.

Declan and I developed a close bond that has continued over the years. I called him by his nickname, *Deco*, and he called me by mine, *Big Al*. We talked about life. We talked about starting a rock band together, with Declan on drums and me as the lead singer. He told me that when he grew up, he either wanted to be a paleontologist or the person who comes into the hospital and plays games with the kids, channeling his dad and his newfound friend, Ed Mckay. He was a cheerful, outgoing child who had a new joke for me almost every time I came to see him:

> "What did one pencil say to the other pencil?"
> "Lookin' sharp!"
>
> "What did the pencil ask another pencil?"
> "What's your point?"
>
> "What did the pencil say to the cowboy?" "Draw!"

The jokes may have been a little corny, but his delivery was exceptional. My responses were just as lame. But unlike Declan, what I lacked in content, I was unable to compensate for in delivery:

> "If you have twelve apples in one hand and eleven pears in the other, what do you have?"
> "Big hands!"
>
> "What did the hat say to the scarf?" "You hang around here. I'll go on ahead!"

The banter sounds inconsequential, but I believe it had a significant effect. It was my attempt to use humor to develop a connection with Declan. By goofing around with him, I was able to earn his trust. And that all-important trust got us through some pretty tough times. The role of a physician is not just to treat but also to heal. The art of healing is to find the correct balance between optimism and reality. Between hope and truth. Sometimes finding that balance is not easy. It means trying to search for some type of silver lining, even when the darkest cloud is overhead. Humor is an underused tool to help find that silver lining.

The importance of humor in healing is underappreciated, particularly when dealing with children. In the words of Victor Borge, "Laughter is the shortest distance between two people." It can be a very effective way to establish and solidify the essential doctor patient relationship. Humor can be a powerful defense mechanism for a fearful child. Norman Cousins wrote eloquently about the role of emotions in health and disease: "Laughter serves as a blocking agent. Like the bulletproof vest, it may help protect you against the ravages of negative emotions that can assault you in disease." The ability to share laughter, particularly with an ailing child, can be a very effective way to build trust.

Declan had turned the corner and was ready to get out of the hospital and go home. His spirits were good and got even better when he learned that on the day of his discharge, the hospital was hosting a parade that featured the real characters from *Star Wars*, Declan's all-time favorite movie. It was an event he will never forget. He got to meet all the actors and then march first in the lineup, carrying the lightsaber of the Jedis while leading the troupe in the parade through the hospital. It was an appropriate sendoff for a remarkable young man.

Children with craniopharyngiomas are patients for life. They often require long-term endocrine monitoring and hormone replacement therapy. They sometimes require repeat surgery and other measures to keep their histologically benign but powerfully forbidding tumor in check. Declan is no exception. We followed him with surveillance MRIs. A year later, he was symptom-free, back in school, and doing well when he had a generalized seizure. A repeat MRI showed recurrence of some of the cystic and solid components of his tumor. The recurrence came from the small scraps we had to leave because they were adherent to the optic nerves and carotid arteries. So, we had to go back to the OR for further decompression surgery.

Once again, we performed an aggressive microsurgical debulking of the tumor. This time, we decided to follow surgery with radiotherapy. Radiation is a treatment usually reserved for cancerous tumors, but it has been found to be effective for selected benign tumors, particularly craniopharyngiomas. Radiation's effectiveness is balanced by its propensity to injure the normal brain as well as the tumor. To mitigate these side effects, we treated Declan with proton beam therapy, which is, in a sense, a gentler form of radiation than conventional photon therapy. Protons are charged particles generated by a cyclotron that deliver a high amount of energy to the tumor but a much lower amount of energy along the trajectory through the brain. Declan received proton beam radiation five days a week for a total of six weeks. The treatments were painless, but for each of the thirty sessions, he had to be put under general anesthesia so he could be perfectly still.

Another setback happened after Declan's tenth radiation treatment. His headaches returned, and an MRI showed marked enlargement of the loculated (non-communicating) tumor cysts at the base of his brain. This didn't come as a surprise—often brain tumor cysts can increase in size transiently during radiotherapy before they shrink once the radiation has done its job. The problem for Declan was that his cysts became very large and symptomatic, causing increased intracranial pressure. So, we decided to interrupt the radiation sessions and operate again, this time using a minimally invasive approach, working through a small exposure with an endoscope to make windows in the cyst walls and allow them to drain into the ventricular system. The procedure worked, and Declan was able to complete his radiation after a week delay. The cysts have not recurred. Neither has the tumor.

That was a tough way for a little five-year-old boy to spend a year of his life. But Declan was resilient and kept a great attitude along the way. Stevi was by his side the entire time. She was distraught throughout the radiotherapy sessions and told Declan she wished she could have been the one put through the treatments instead of him. "Don't worry, Mom," Declan told Stevi. "I can do this. I would never want to put you through it." It made me realize that in some ways, Declan was as strong and *adamantinomatous* as his tumor. He spent the early part of his life undergoing multiple brain surgeries and radiation therapy, but he was unbreakable. He would not allow this treacherous growth at the base of his brain get the better of him. As is often the case in dealing with pediatric brain tumors, I find that the strength of the child can help the rest of the family get through the experience.

Declan has been clinically stable for the past several years, with no evidence of recurrence of his craniopharyngioma. At the time of this writing, he is a typical thirteen-year-old boy in the eighth grade. His favorite class is math. He had a relaxing summer going to the pool and hanging out with friends. He and his family had a great family visit to Disney World. They are planning a family trip to Ireland.

Now that Declan is in middle school, his parents got him a cell phone, and he has created a chat group with six of his friends so that they can text one another. He also uses his phone to play a variety of online games, including Cookie Clicker, Fruit Ninja, Marvel Strike Force, and Dragon Ball. His favorite subject in school is math, and among other subjects, he will be studying Chinese this year. He continues to fight with his nine-year-old brother, Oliver, calling him "a jerk who gets on my nerves." In his spare time, Declan helps the family care for their two dogs, both pugs, Mabel, age twelve weeks and the runt of the litter, and Pepper, age five years.

As an academic pediatric neurosurgeon, I have also relied on humor in my role as an educator. The molecular biology of pediatric brain tumors can get pretty dense. It can be difficult to hold the attention of the medical school class in lectures and prevent them from surreptitiously using their laptops or cell phones to answer emails and texts. So, to prevent that from happening, I wrote a song about craniopharyngioma, hoping it would pique the interest of the medical students and inspire them to read more about the topic. It was a country and western tune, set to the background music of the classic, "Cryin' Time." I called it, "Extreme Craniopharyngioma."

As it happened, around the time I wrote the song, the Pediatric Section of the American Association of Neurological Surgeons and Congress of Neurological Surgeons held its annual meeting in Cleveland, Ohio, the city where I was working at the time. The banquet was being held at the Rock and Roll Hall of Fame, and live music was provided by a local country and western band. I thought this would be a good opportunity for me to reach a new audience, so I approached the band, gave them a copy of what I felt were my classic lyrics, and asked if they would back me up while I sang it to my peers. To my surprise, they said, "Sure, no problem. We've got your back."

That's all I needed to hear. That's how I found myself on stage at the Rock and Roll Hall of Fame, making my debut while the audience was having their dessert. With apologies to Tammy Wynette and George Jones, here's a sample:

Cranio pharyngioma you're so hateful,

You're the most forbidding tumor in the brain,

When I peel you off the stalk, I feel so grateful,

Please don't come back, or I will surely go insane.

The backup band was terrific, and for me, it was the experience of a lifetime. But I'll never forget the words of Sunil Manjila, my neurosurgery resident, who was in the audience, sitting right next to the platform. He approached me as I was leaving the stage: "Al, I don't understand what just happened. How did you do that? You got a standing ovation from the audience, and you couldn't even sing on key." At that point, still riding the wave of success, I looked Sunil in the eye and repeated the words inscribed on my residency graduation plaque: *Melior fortunas quam bonus esse* ("It's better to be lucky than good").

Years have passed, and to look at Declan today, you would not be able to recognize the ordeal he had gone through. His hair has grown back, and he's a normal kid. Even his height, which was one of the issues that brought him to medical attention in the first place, is no longer a problem. The endocrinology team began him on somatropin, a recombinant form of human growth hormone replacement, after he completed his proton beam radiation. His height has normalized. The medication has to be administered carefully because of concern that in addition to helping Declan grow, it could promote growth of any residual tumor. Fortunately, careful follow-up with surveillance MRIs has shown no evidence of any tumor recurrence. Dr. Mike Repka of ophthalmology has been following Declan over the years, and his eye exam has been normal.

Declan and I still talk from time to time. The jokes haven't gotten any better, but the connection is still rock solid.

CHAPTER 8

Denial

"Denial is the way we handle what we can't handle."

Anonymous

For Jami Carr, Friday, July 7, 2023, began pretty much just like any other day. The only difference was that she didn't sleep well the night before, lying awake for hours with anxiety about her eleven-year-old daughter, Charlotte, who was scheduled to have some blood work done that morning. Charlotte had been having headaches and nausea for the past couple of weeks and wasn't bouncing back. Her pediatrician had ordered the blood tests.

Charlotte, who went by the nickname Charli, was deathly afraid of needles, and Jami was apprehensive that she would have to endure something that was so scary to her. Would she cry? Would she faint? Would she be okay? At the time, Jami had no idea that the events of the next twenty-four hours would turn her life upside down, along with the lives of her daughter and her entire family.

The Carrs were a happy family of five. Jami worked as the director of admissions at St. Mary's School in Annapolis, Maryland, and her husband Taylor was a business technology executive. They had three daughters. Charli was the middle child, between her older sister Duffy (age twelve) and younger sister Mary (age six). They had recently returned from a weeklong vacation on the ocean at Rehoboth, Delaware. Jami had the day off to take Charli for the blood tests.

To quiet her anxiety, Jami immersed herself in the morning's activities. She made breakfast for the family, did laundry, and got the girls' equipment ready for horseback riding camp at the Oak Crest Riding Farm in Harwood, Maryland. Horseback riding was a favorite activity of the girls, and this was the final day of horseback riding camp. It was a special camp that they had looked forward to joining for several years, and this year, they were finally granted a spot. Charli was an avid rider. Her favorite horse was an old brown mare named Mocha. But this Friday, only two of the three girls would be going. Charli had no interest in camp this morning. She was too tired. It was too hot outside. Her head hurt. In retrospect, Jami realized that was all part of a bigger problem.

So, Jami helped get Duffy and Mary dressed and prepared to drop them off at camp. She decided to let Charli sleep in. Taylor was working at home and would keep an eye on her. Charli had gone to bed very nervous about the needle. Jami felt the more her daughter slept, the less time she'd have to stress over the blood work.

When Jami returned home, Charli was already awake, and they drove to Labcorp at Walgreens for the blood tests. They had to wait for about twenty minutes before Charli was called in, but she was doing okay, and the women were very nice and did a wonderful job keeping her relaxed while they drew her blood. Charli felt a little lightheaded afterward, so she sat in a chair for fifteen minutes while Jami brought her some juice and took her to get a strawberry banana smoothie, her favorite. Charli felt much better after the smoothie and was very proud of herself. They phoned her grandparents from the car on the way home to tell them how brave she was.

Charli had been in her usual state of good health until two weeks earlier, when, on Saturday morning, June 24, she was participating in a swim meet doing the backstroke and struck the back of her head against the wall of the pool when she was turning. She felt dazed but didn't lose consciousness. Jami took her home and noticed that she didn't have much of an appetite that day. Charli went to bed early that night and awoke with pretty bad headache, which continued throughout the day. Jami and Taylor suspected she had sustained a concussion from her head injury in the pool the day before.

That weekend, the family set off for their planned weeklong vacation at the beach in Rehoboth, Delaware. The weather was great, but Charli continued to feel sick each day, with a persistent diffuse headache, for which she took Tylenol without significant relief. They returned home the following Saturday. When Charli got out of the car, she said, "I feel really lousy."

Jami was upset and snapped at Charli, believing she was acting out. She felt that after a week, the symptoms of a concussion should be getting better. She told Charli to go lie down in her bedroom. When Charli reached her bedroom, the headache worsened, and she vomited profusely. Jami now realized that something was wrong, apologized for her behavior, and brought Charli to the local urgent care center the next day, a Sunday. Charli had a low-grade fever, but her exam was okay otherwise. She hadn't been eating well and had lost some weight. They tested her for COVID-19, streptococcus, and influenza. All studies were negative. The physician thought she had a viral illness and suggested that she go home and take it easy for the next few days. Jami knew there was a virus going around and took Charli home to rest. Common things are common, she thought. It must be a virus.

Charli just hung around at home for the next few days, not doing much. She laid on the couch complaining that she was exhausted and had a headache. On Wednesday, she had another episode of profuse emesis. Now Jami and Taylor became seriously concerned. There must be something else going on, they thought.

The next morning, Jami called their pediatrician, Dr. Faith Hackett, and conveyed her concerns about Charli. Dr. Hackett arranged for an urgent visit that afternoon. She saw that Charli was tired and pale. She thought Charli might have been dehydrated from a virus. Or maybe she was anemic. She wondered whether Charli could have Lyme disease. Lyme disease is a tick-borne illness caused by the bacterium *Borrelia burgdorferi*. It is transmitted to humans by the bite of an infected black-legged tick, also known as the deer tick. Early symptoms include fever, a characteristic circular "bull's eye" rash called erythema migrans, fatigue, muscle aches, and headache.

Dr. Hackett noted that Charli did have many of the symptoms of early Lyme disease, and even though she didn't appear to have a rash, the Carrs did live out in the country, where Charli could have been exposed to ticks. So, Dr. Hackett set up a series of blood tests for the next day, including a complete blood count, electrolytes, a viral panel, and an immunological test for Lyme disease. She told Charli to go home and hydrate, which she did, and she actually began to feel a little better.

Jami started spinning about Lyme disease. She didn't know a lot about the disorder, but she knew enough to realize that it could be serious, with lifelong consequences. Jami told her mother, "I keep thinking how sad I will be if a stupid tick bite might be the cause of devastating lifetime consequences."

The routine blood work on Friday morning, July 7, that Dr. Hackett had ordered came back normal. As Jami was driving Charli home, she was talking on the cell phone to Charli's grandfather, letting him know how well Charli had done. As soon as they hung up, Jami got a phone call from Dr. Hackett. Dr. Hackett told her that she had struggled to sleep the night before. She said, "I know Charli, and I know you. This is not in character for her." She said she didn't want to be an alarmist and cause any unnecessary stress, but that she would feel more comfortable if they could get Charli an MRI of her head, in that it was already Friday with the weekend approaching. "I just want to dot our i's and cross our "t's," she said. Jami agreed.

So, Jami went home and tried to schedule the MRI, but the next available appointment was in three weeks. Dr. Hackett phoned in a request for an emergency scan that day. Fortunately, there was a cancellation, and Charli got an appointment for 3:30 p.m. later that afternoon. It was the last scan of the day. Jami remembers the MRI tech being somewhat brusque and impatient with them, trying to move things along quickly.

Charli was stoic and got through the entire scan without any problem. She even slept through part of it. Jami sat with her in the scanner and wondered how Charli could do so well because the machine made so much noise.

At the end of the scan, the technician returned and seemed like a completely different person—kind, caring, and soft-spoken. At the time, Jami never even considered that he had likely looked at the images before he returned. Jami took Charli directly home and promised her that she could take a bath, put on some cozy pajamas, and have a relaxed weekend. She promised Charli that by Monday, she would be all better.

An hour later, the phone rang. It was Dr. Hackett calling from her mobile phone—not her office. Jami closed her bedroom door, and she remembers thinking that it was odd for her to do so. What could Dr. Hackett possibly have to say that I would not want my children to see or hear my reaction to? Dr. Hackett said she was so very sorry and asked if Jami's husband was home. Jami told her he wouldn't be back for another hour or so. She told Jami to sit down. She said, "I don't even know how to say this. The MRI showed a mass in the center of Charli's brain. She has a brain tumor and hydrocephalus. I'm so sorry to give you this news."

Dr. Hackett told Jami to call her parents, who lived just down the street, to come right over and watch Charli's sisters. She told Jami to pack a bag and drive directly to Johns Hopkins Medical Center. Jami remembers a feeling of panic as she repeated that she didn't know what to do or even how to get to Johns Hopkins. Dr. Hackett told her to just get Charli in the car and start driving. She would give her directions. She told Jami how much she loved her and Charli and that she would be with them every step of the way. Jami remembered hearing that as she was holding back tears. This was the first moment it dawned on her that if these results were correct, her daughter was severely ill, and there was nothing she could do about it.

But that couldn't be the case, she thought. She knew Charli would be okay. This stuff happened in the movies. It happened to other families. Not hers. Somehow during that time of packing and getting into the car, a total of five minutes, she convinced herself that the MRI was wrong. A mistake had been made. Everything was going to be alright.

The drive to the Hopkins Emergency Room took an hour, and Jami doesn't remember most of it. The only thing she does remember is her husband calling her and telling her he was on his way to meet them. He asked her what the MRI showed, and she told him she couldn't say it out loud. "I was petrified to put these words into the universe," she said, "to give them life, to allow them to come true. This was not her story. Not us. Not our child."

She held Charli's hand as they drove. She told Charli that they would go to Hopkins, where they would take a new picture of her brain. "They will tell us it was a mistake and send us home. I am certain."

Initially, things moved quickly in the ER. They called Charli's name after about a ten-minute wait and put her in a room, took her vital signs, asked about her symptoms and examined her. She had grade 2 papilledema, swelling of the optic discs resulting from increased intracranial pressure.

Charli was moved from the ER to the Pediatric Intensive Care Unit at 1 a.m. and was scheduled for a high-resolution MRI of her brain and spine at 3:30 a.m. Jami recalls, "Again, I sat at her feet during the MRI. It was the first time I cried. I cried for my baby. I prayed this was, in fact, a big mistake. I begged God to make it me and not her. I felt I was hanging from a cliff and someone else had my hands. At any time, they could let me go. It was all out of my control. It was the worst feeling any parent could have."

I met Jami Carr for the first time at 5:30 a.m. on Saturday, July 8, 2023. The MRI had just finished, and Charli was being whisked back to the PICU. I was making rounds with my team when we ran into Jami in the Radiology Suite, where the MRI had been done. We had seen the scan even before we had a chance to examine Charli.

I showed Jami the MRI on a computer console in the room. "There's a large tumor deep in her brain," I said, pointing to the mass filling the frontal horn of the left lateral ventricle. "It's blocking the outflow of cerebrospinal fluid from the ventricles on both sides, causing hydrocephalus and increased pressure inside her head. This is what's causing her symptoms. There are also several smaller tumors deep in the brain, but they don't appear to be causing a problem. When we see multiple tumors in the brain, it is serious and can mean they are malignant, a form of brain cancer. But there is hope," I continued, "because some of the imaging characteristics suggest the lesions may be low-grade and slow-growing, that is, not cancer. And the MRI of the spine is completely normal."

This is the challenge of balancing honesty with hope. Here I was, a complete stranger, telling a mother that her precious, beloved child had a large symptomatic brain tumor that would require urgent surgery. Jami would tell me later that I was the bearer of the worst news she had ever received in her life. The previous MRI was not a mistake. The tumor was real. But I was cautiously optimistic that we could get Charli safely through the surgery and return her to her normal life. The art of healing is always a delicate balance between honesty and hope. There is no one-size-fits-all solution, but it is important to find something positive to say, even when one is delivering news that is not good.

For Jami, this was still a devastating blow. And her initial response of denial is something we all experience as a method of defense. The Swiss American psychiatrist Elisabeth Kubler-Ross said, "Denial helps us to pace our feelings of grief. There is a grace in denial. It is nature's way of letting in only as much as we can handle." As Jami began to accept the harsh reality of the circumstances, she became a fierce advocate for her daughter, helping her and the rest of the family navigate the terrifying days to come.

We placed Charli on a steroid, dexamethasone, to reduce the swelling in her head and an anti-seizure medication, levetiracetam. We broke the rules and allowed Charli's sisters and other family members including her Aunt Lisa, who works in Radiology at Johns Hopkins, to come into the PICU to have a party. We reviewed her MRI in detail and kept an eye on her in the PICU over the weekend with plans to remove the tumor on Monday.

The MRI showed a large contrast-enhancing suprasellar tumor above the pituitary gland, deep in the brain, extending upward into the frontal horn of the left lateral ventricle, abutting the midline ventricular septum pellucidum that separates the two lateral ventricles. The tumor pushed the septum over to the right and obstructed both foramina of Monro, drainage passages within the ventricles, causing a backup of cerebrospinal fluid thereby creating hydrocephalus and increased intracranial pressure. Inferiorly, the tumor appeared to arise from the hypothalamus, the master gland that regulates hormonal secretion. There were two smaller tumors in the parahippocampal gyri, which play a role in memory encoding and retrieval, at the medial border of the temporal lobes. Another small mass was seen deep in the right side of the brain in the thalamus. None of the tumors restricted diffusion, and they all had imaging characteristics suggesting that they might be low grade, even though they were in several different locations.

We focused on the large intraventricular mass. That's where the problem was. Although the tumor involved the hypothalamus, the endocrine team felt she was stable, and all of her endocrine labs were normal. We needed to make a tissue diagnosis and remove as much of the tumor as we safely could, in order to open up the ventricular system and allow the cerebrospinal fluid to flow freely again.

On Monday morning, at the crack of dawn, Jami and Taylor tearfully said goodbye to their sweet, brave daughter as she was wheeled off to the OR, not knowing what kind of condition she would be in when they saw her again.

I was fortunate to be operating with two tremendous assistant neurosurgeons, Rachel Pruitt and Connor Liu. We positioned Charli supine on the OR table and proceeded to go after the tumor. We had planned the procedure carefully and set out to perform a left frontal craniotomy. We used frameless stereotactic navigation based on Charli's preoperative MRI to choose the optimal corridor to take us to the tumor. The approach was also facilitated by the use of transdural ultrasonography (sonar) to precisely localize the tumor's margins. We carried out the resection through a small corridor, working under the guidance of the operating microscope. The tumor appeared grayish white, moderately tough in consistency, but myxoid (mucinous) and suctionable. We were able to resect the tumor and unblock the foramina of Monro, effectively treating her hydrocephalus.

Frozen section pathology returned consistent with a glial neoplasm with myxomatous changes. That's all we needed to hear. It confirmed our own pre-op and intra-op suspicions that this was a low-grade, non-cancerous glial tumor. We closed up, leaving a temporary drain in the ventricle of the brain for forty-eight hours to clean out any blood products and debris.

Eight hours after we had started the case, I went to see Jami and Taylor in the waiting room. They both appeared ashen. They both considered it the longest day of their lives. It's a response that is all too common. Jami was clearly beside herself. She had paced the floors of the hospital the entire time. Later she told me, "I prayed more during those eight hours than I ever did in two years of Catholic school combined. I prayed that God would give Charli back to me. If she couldn't walk, I would carry her. I just wanted her back in any shape or form that God would give her to me."

I spoke to Jami and Taylor for a good ten minutes, recounting everything we did in the OR. Later Jami would tell me, "I don't remember a single word you said except your first sentence: 'She did great.'" But that was all she needed to hear. At that moment, she felt that she was finally able to get back on her feet again after the longest cliff fall of her life. It is a curious but common phenomenon for families not to register much of what is said in the debriefing in the recovery room after a loved one has undergone major surgery. Emotions run strong, and conversations often need to be repeated before the meaning sets in. But this time, the news was good.

We went to the bedside to see Charli. She was extubated with her eyes open, looking around at us and tracking us with her eyes. We had placed a white turban headwrap on her head in the shape of a shark—she had told us she loved sharks, and her favorite stuffed animal was a shark. She looked like a real ICU patient—she had a lot of tubes coming out of her, including two IVs, an arterial line, a catheter in her bladder, and a ventricular drain coming out of her head. She was starting to follow commands but did not speak yet and had significant weakness of her right arm and leg, the opposite side where we had operated. And she had a large emesis in the presence of her family.

Maybe I shouldn't have been so optimistic when speaking to the family, I thought. It's always safer to underpromise and overdeliver. But the operation had gone so well, and the brain had looked so good as we closed. Sometimes it takes a while for the anesthesia to wear off. "Let's give her a little more time to come around," I said, somewhat cautiously.

Fortunately, Charli came around quickly. She started speaking. Her first word was "Mommy," and she began talking in full sentences. Her right hemiparesis resolved, and she was able to lift all extremities off the bed. Her MRI looked good, showing post-operative changes with resection of the ventricular tumor and reduction in size of her ventricles, which had become unblocked. The three very small, deep-seated tumors adjacent to her brainstem that we left alone were unchanged. Two days later, we were able to remove Charli's ventricular drain and all of her lines and transfer her up to the regular floor. She had no more vomiting, and her eating improved.

As a young girl, she was concerned about her appearance, with a seventeen-centimeter scar across the top of her head. "What am I gonna tell people?" she asked, a bit anxiously.

"Don't worry, Charli, the hair will grow back and hide the incision," I told her.

"But what will I tell them now, before my hair grows back?" she asked.

"Why don't you figure something out and have fun with it?" I said, conspiring with her. "Clearly, you like sharks. Make up a good story. Tell people you were attacked by a shark while swimming at the beach. Why not?"

And that's exactly what she did, with a sparkle in her beautiful brown eyes, both in the hospital and when she went back to classes in the sixth grade in middle school. She held her head high and wore her hair short in a buzz cut and didn't hide her incision, even on class picture day. Her classmates and teachers were all extremely supportive. And to seal the deal she wore a T-shirt for weeks that said, SHARK ATTACK SURVIVOR.

The pathology report returned pilomyxoid astrocytoma. The name comes from Greek (*pilo*, "hair," and *myxoid*, "resembling slime, mucus"). The pilomyxoid astrocytoma is a low-grade tumor first described in 1999 by the brilliant Johns Hopkins neuropathologist, Peter Burger in the *Journal of Neuropathology & Experimental Neurology*. The pilomyxoid astrocytoma is a variant of the pilocytic astrocytoma, the most common primary brain tumor of childhood, considered to be benign based on its indolent behavior.

When we remove a low-grade brain tumor from a child, we often follow a course of watchful waiting, using the child's clinical course and surveillance MR imaging to make sure things remain stable. But Charli's case was a little different, because we had noted three other small, deeply situated tumors on her preoperative MRI, two in the parahippocampal gyri of the medial temporal lobes (one on the right and one on the left) and another in the right thalamus. Most of the time when there are multiple tumors in the brain, it means the tumor is malignant and has spread. But there are cases of low-grade indolent tumors that are multi-focal. And the question is how best to manage them.

The first issue is to ask whether the three small shadows we see on the MRI are really tumors. There's no way to know for sure without removing them and sending specimens to the neuropathologist to make a definitive diagnosis. We suspected that they were tumors because their imaging appearance on MRI is so similar to the ventricular tumor we removed. We could operate and remove each of the smaller tumors, but because of their deep location, that approach would create a risk of causing injury to the brain in the approach for the resection. And the tumors hadn't changed in size during our short period of observation.

In this case, we chose to monitor her satellite lesions with surveillance MRIs. We crave certainty in medicine, but things are rarely there in black and white. It was most likely that the shadows on Charli's MRI were low-grade tumors, the same type as the one we removed. But sometimes these lesions can remain unchanged and even undergo senescence and shrink. We'll back off on the frequency of the scans if the shadows remain stable, and we're prepared to treat them if they grow.

Charli was discharged from the hospital in good condition. Her headache was gone, and she had no further vomiting. Her right-sided weakness had gone away. An outpatient visit to the ophthalmologist confirmed that her papilledema had resolved. Repeat MRI showed no further hydrocephalus now that the large tumor blocking the ventricles had been removed.

But there was another issue to deal with—those blood tests ordered by Dr. Hackett. The routine studies had come back normal, but the immunoglobulin test for Lyme disease ultimately returned positive. Charli did live in a rural area endemic for Lyme disease. And she had a constellation of symptoms compatible with Lyme disease. Yet we were certain that her signs and symptoms of increased intracranial pressure were due to the large intraventricular brain tumor and hydrocephalus. And we knew that these resolved after the brain tumor was resected. We consulted Dr. Aaron Milstone of the Infectious Diseases department, who felt that it was unlikely that Charli had active Lyme disease. But he recommended that we treat her for Lyme disease to eliminate any possibility that this could have contributed in any way to her illness. So, we gave Charli a fourteen-day course of the antibiotic, doxycycline, which she tolerated without any problem.

To help Charli through her ordeal, Jami and Taylor got her an enormous Mastiff puppy, who weighed forty pounds at age fifteen weeks. Pets can provide substantial comfort for children as well as adults who are struggling with illness. I remember in the early years of my career, I had a Newfoundland named Morty, a "gentle giant" who weighed 190 pounds. One sunny hot spring Sunday, I brought Morty to a canine carnival being held at Chagrin Falls, a lovely rural suburb of Cleveland. There must have been several hundred people at the event with their pets. There were lots of activities for families and kids. And there were loads of booths with vendors selling toys and supplies for all the pets. Everyone seemed to be having fun.

I was standing next to a large above-ground kiddie pool that had been set up to allow the dogs to come over and have a drink of water. That's what several of them were doing as I turned my head and noticed that when I wasn't looking, my Morty had walked into the center of the kiddie pool to lift up his leg and pee in it in front of everyone. I was dumbfounded with embarrassment and carefully pulled on the leash to get Morty out of the pool so that I could walk away with him, pretending that I didn't realize what had transpired. Pets are wonderful, but sometimes, they come with baggage.

It has now been three years since Charli's brain tumor surgery. She's a happy healthy kid back in school. She plays and jokes and runs around with her friends. She went to the Horizon Survivor's Day Camp at the St. Timothy School over the summer. It's a great camp for kids and their siblings who've been through a tough time. And it's free.

Charli just got a pair of gray rubber shark flip-flops to make a new fashion statement. She celebrated Shark Week this year by wearing her new shark shoes and her old shark shirt. In spite of her concussive head injury last year, she's back on the swimming team. And she's been saddling up for horseback rides on her beloved Mocha. She is asymptomatic and is on no medications. We are following her with no adjuvant treatment. Her surveillance MRI two years following surgery shows no recurrence of the tumor. Her brain looks great.

For me, things have come full circle now because Charli has granted me the ultimate honor, naming her one-year-old giant Mastiff, currently 160 pounds, Maggie *Cohen* Carr. The name may not roll easily off the tongue, but who am I to complain?

CHAPTER 9

Sweet Angel

"It is so much darker when a light goes out than it would have been if it had never shone."

John Steinbeck
The Winter of Our Discontent

For thirty-eight-year-old Rene Marsh, Thursday, March 14, 2019, was the best day of her life. At 5:30 a.m., the newborn nursery nurse handed Rene her first-born child, a beautiful boy named Blake. He was a full-term baby, born via normal spontaneous vaginal delivery at the Virginia Hospital Center. He weighed six pounds, five ounces. "It was as if she handed me my heart," she said.

As Rene cradled him in her arms for the first time, she remembers a single tear falling from her eye to her cheek as she was bursting with the joy of becoming a mother. She was overcome with a sense of deep pure love that she had never before experienced. She and her husband, Kedric Payne, brought Blake home, where he was adored by family and friends and brought happiness to everyone around him with his radiant smile and extroverted personality.

Nine months after Blake was born, the same amount of time Rene carried him in her womb, I met with Rene and Kedric early in the morning on Christmas Eve in Blake's room on the pediatric floor of Johns Hopkins Hospital. Blake had just undergone an MRI examination of his brain. I had the agonizing task of bringing them the worst news they had ever heard in their lives.

Rene and Kedric were a storybook couple. Kedric first noticed Rene in 2014 at the Alfred Street Baptist Church in Alexandria, Virginia, but they didn't have an opportunity to talk to one another. They met later in the week at a dance party at the iconic Howard Theatre on T Street in Washington, DC, and began dating. They were married in November 2017 at a private ceremony at the Morais Vineyards and Winery in Bealeton, Virginia. The wedding was carefully choreographed, with Rene walking down the aisle to John Legend's "All of Me."

Rene was born in Brooklyn, New York, to Jamaican parents who immigrated to the United States in the 1960s. She grew up in Queens and earned a bachelor's degree in English with honors at Binghamton University. She went on to earn a master's degree in broadcast journalism from the S.I. Newhouse School of Public Communication at Syracuse University. After several jobs in journalism, Rene joined CNN in 2012, where she works as an Emmy-nominated national correspondent in its Washington Bureau.

Kedric was born in Memphis, Tennessee, and earned a bachelor of arts degree in political science with honors at Yale and a law degree from the University of Pennsylvania, where he served as editor in chief of the *Law Review*. Early in his career, he worked as a court law clerk for the Southern District of New

York. He is currently the vice president, general counsel, and senior director of ethics at the nonpartisan Campaign Legal Center in Washington, DC.

As soon as Blake was born, he became the center of attention for Rene and Kedric. They affectionately nicknamed him "Blakey," and he was the perfect child, the epitome of health. Rene called him her *sweet angel.* From the day he was born, Blakey was the star, and everything else revolved around him. He was a charmer and brought laughter to every room he was in. He loved hugging and kissing and throwing all his toys on the floor. He loved being read to and was passionate about music, particularly Mozart. Life was perfect.

One day in late November 2019, when Blakey was nine months old, Rene noted that he appeared cross-eyed. His left eye was turned in. He had received a flu shot two weeks earlier but otherwise had been fine. She brought him to see an ophthalmologist, who diagnosed strabismus (Greek: *strabismus,* "squinting"). Strabismus is a condition in which the eyes are misaligned. The ophthalmologist performed a dilated eye exam that was normal. Normally the six muscles attached to each eye are yoked and move the eyes together, but Blakey's eyes weren't properly aligned. He had an esotropia of the left eye, meaning that it was turned inward. Strabismus is a relatively common problem, and the ophthalmologist recommended a regimen of ocular patching of the right eye to increase the strength of the lateral rectus muscle that moves the left eye outward. It didn't work.

On December 22, Blakey still had a left esotropia despite the patching, and now the eye was tearing, and the eyelid was swollen. That was all that was wrong with him. He was otherwise fine. Rene and Kedric brought him to the Johns Hopkins Hospital Emergency Room, where he was examined by one of the ophthalmologists from the world-class Wilmer Eye Clinic at Hopkins. The ophthalmologist was concerned about a left abducens nerve palsy and the possibility of an orbital mass. The abducens nerve is the sixth cranial nerve, whose purpose is to innervate the left lateral rectus muscle of the eye and abduct it, that is, turn it outward. The ophthalmologist ordered an MRI of the orbits and the brain. To get this done, Blakey would have to be placed under general anesthesia so that he would hold still for the study. So, he was admitted to the pediatric service at Johns Hopkins.

The MRI was performed without any problem. There was no mass in the orbit. But to everyone's surprise, there was a large, solid, contrast-enhancing, lobular tumor in the midline at the base of the brain. It was in the suprasellar area, just above the pituitary gland. It looked angry. The tumor spilled over and eroded into the cavernous sinuses on each side. The cavernous sinuses are trabeculous (partitioned) channels that lie within a splitting of the dura mater, the fibrous lining of the brain, at the base of the skull on either side of the bony sella turcica (Latin for "Turkish saddle"), the seat of the pituitary gland. The cavernous sinuses contain some important structures, including the internal carotid arteries and several of the cranial nerves (the oculomotor, trochlear, trigeminal, and abducens), which arise from the brainstem and innervate the face and eyes.

The tumor had destroyed a portion of the clivus (Latin for "slope"), the bone at the skull base on which the brainstem rests. It compressed the optic nerves upward and displaced the brainstem backward and pushed the pituitary gland downward. It exhibited restriction of diffusion which, in this setting, was suggestive of a malignant tumor, a brain cancer. An MRI of the spine was performed to ensure that there was no spread of disease outside the brain. The spine MRI was normal. A CT scan of the brain was performed to help delineate the nature of the tumor and the surrounding skull base. The CT showed heavy calcification at the top of the tumor.

So that was the state of things on Tuesday, December 24, 2019, Christmas Eve morning, as I went to meet with Rene and Kedric for the first time to discuss these formidable findings and make a plan. I had already spent several hours discussing the case with my colleagues in pediatric neurosurgery. I sought advice from my partners at Johns Hopkins and from my associates across the country. I also consulted with Hopkins colleagues in oncology, neurology, neuroradiology, endocrinology, and anesthesiology. Here was a nine-month-old infant boy who looked perfectly fine except his left eye was turned inward. The left-sided periorbital swelling had somehow resolved on its own. But we had the surprise finding on MRI of a monster tumor deep in the center of his brain.

There was no consensus about what type of tumor this was. One of the neuroradiologists wondered if it could be an atypical craniopharyngioma, a benign tumor, because of its location, geometry, and calcification. Calcification can sometimes, but not always, suggest a more benign process, and pediatric craniopharyngiomas often have calcification. But other characteristics on the MRI, such as the tumor's invasiveness and diffusion restriction, made it appear to be more malignant, likely some type of primitive embryonal tumor, an aggressive brain cancer.

Blakey would need surgery to enable us to make a tissue diagnosis and remove as much tumor as was safely possible. The location of the tumor, deep in the center of the brain, gave us some concern about how best to plan the surgical approach. Sometimes we can get to this area by going through the nose, a transsphenoidal corridor, the same way most pituitary tumors in adults are removed. But Blakey was very young, and his cranial sinuses were too small to work through. In addition, his pituitary gland, the pea-sized endocrine gland, was functioning normally and was in the way. He would require a craniotomy.

I steeled myself as I sat down in Blakey's hospital room to talk with Rene and Kedric. I showed them the MRI on the computer screen. "Blakey has a large aggressive tumor growing at the base of his brain," I said. "I think it's malignant, likely a form of brain cancer. We will need to operate to find out what it is and remove as much as we safely can. We will need to perform a craniotomy, temporarily removing a piece of his skull on the right side of his head, then working under the microscope, lifting up the brain and working through a small space underneath it, to get to the tumor."

I went on and explained more details about how we would do the surgery and discussed the surgical risks we would have to deal with. The room fell silent. Giving news like this is one of the most unpleasant tasks I have ever done. It is the worst part of my job. There is no way for a family to prepare for what they are about to hear. Their beautiful precious baby has a cancerous growth in the center of his brain. How can they even process what they hear?

I sensed that after my first sentence about the large aggressive brain tumor, much of what I said was not processed. This is often the case I encounter when breaking bad news to patients and families. This is true even for medically sophisticated families. They go into a state of shock. There is no easy way to deliver news like this. Things I have found to be helpful are to be honest but compassionate, to be patient and give time for words to sink in, to sit with the family allowing for silence, answer questions as they come up, to be empathetic, and to always offer some form of hope. That doesn't mean to sugarcoat the situation. But even in dire circumstances, it is important to introduce some form of hope. Where there is life, there's hope.

"We'll get Blakey ready and do the surgery the day after tomorrow," I said. "And we'll be here with you each day to help get you through this. Our goal is to get the surgery safely behind us. I suggest trying to break things up into manageable chunks. One day at a time."

I placed a pen mark on the right side of Blakey's head. It's the simple things that can get a surgeon into big trouble, like operating on the wrong side of the head. I went through the routine risks, benefits, and alternatives and obtained informed consent for the surgery,

Kedric later told me that he was initially overcome with fear but managed to pull himself together by turning inward to his deep religious faith, which helped give him courage to push on. Rene would later tell me she felt as if the lights went out in the room and the floor underneath her gave way. She had an intense feeling of fright and pain, as if she was falling from a thirteen-story building, except she was sitting in the room, completely still. She felt a strong heaviness in her chest. It was like a horrible nightmare, only worse, because she couldn't wake up from it.

We operated on little Blakey two days later, on Thursday, December 26, the day after Christmas. Rene and Kedric accompanied him to the OR. Blakey loved music, and he was particularly fond of Bob Marley and the Wailers. So, with Blakey on the OR table and the anesthesia team gently putting him under, we played "Three Little Birds" on the stereo. It's a beautiful, melodic, calming song. One of the OR nurses quietly ushered

Rene and Kedric to the waiting room, as they left their brave little boy in our hands to probe the depths of his brain. There wasn't a dry eye in the OR.

I performed the surgery with Andrew Kobets, my extremely bright and capable fellow at the time. The first thing we did was to perform a lumbar puncture, a spinal tap, to remove some cerebrospinal fluid in order to relax the brain for the surgery to come. We also sent some of the fluid for tumor markers and cytopathologic analysis. We had sent some bloodwork for tumor markers earlier, in the hope of finding a clue about the nature of the tumor, but the bloodwork was normal. Often for a surgery like Blakey's, we leave a spinal catheter in place during the operation to keep the brain relaxed. But in this case, we didn't feel that was safe to do, because Blakey was so small. Instead, we sieved the dura at the site of the lumbar puncture, hoping the multiple small punctures in the dura would enable some cerebrospinal fluid to leak into the muscles of his back and relax the brain.

Next, with Blakey's little head turned to the left and supported on a padded horseshoe headrest, we performed a right-sided orbitozygomatic craniotomy to enable us to gently elevate the brain and work through a narrow corridor underneath it in order to reach the deep-seated tumor. In this type of exposure, our craniotomy involved removing some of the frontal and temporal bones at the base of the skull, along with the zygoma (cheekbone) and a portion of the orbit, all of which we replace at the end of the surgery. This exposure allows us to minimize the amount of retraction we have to use to reach the tumor. We also used an electromagnetic image guidance system with a probe that acted like a magic wand, a sort of neurosurgical GPS technique, so that we could reach the tumor using the safest corridor.

Under magnification provided by the operating microscope, we found the tumor, which was grayish, firm, gritty, and vascular, and we began to remove it. It did not come easily, but we used a variety of microsurgical instruments and removed a large amount of tumor. We stopped short of removing the entire tumor for fear of tearing its attachment to the cavernous sinus on each side and causing catastrophic bleeding or injury to the adjacent cranial nerves. We controlled bleeding from the tumor bed and closed up in routine fashion. Usually, we replace the bone flap with titanium microplates and screws, but because Blakey was so young, we secured the bone with low-profile absorbable plates and screws that dissolve over time. The operation took just under seven hours.

Blakey woke up nicely after the operation and was extubated. We brought him back to his bed in the PICU.

The tumor had been sent to pathology. The frozen section biopsy returned while we were in the OR as a hypercellular small round blue cell tumor with brisk mitotic activity (cellular division) under light microscopy. There was evidence of necrosis (cell death) along with Homer Wright rosettes and Flexner-Wintersteiner rosettes (groups of tumor cells arranged in a pattern resembling a rose).

This confirmed our clinical suspicion in the OR. The tumor was definitely not a benign craniopharyngioma. It was an aggressive malignant tumor, brain cancer, likely some type of primitive high-grade central nervous system embryonal tumor, arising from cells left over from fetal development in the womb. More tumor specimens were sent for special stains and molecular analysis.

I went to talk to Rene and Kedric in the waiting room. Their long hours of waiting during the surgery had been excruciating. They tried to distract themselves with a little levity by watching clips of *Saturday Night Live* sketches on Kedric's iPad. But their anxiety level was high, and the humor fell short.

"The surgery went well," I said. "We were able to get a good resection of the tumor, and Blakey is already waking up nicely from surgery. Unfortunately, the biopsy confirmed our worst suspicion. It looks like an embryonal tumor, which is an aggressive form of brain cancer. Blakey will need further treatment with chemotherapy to help control the tumor. But right now, we want to focus on letting him recover from the surgery, and the good news is that he's recovering very nicely."

Silence once again. Kedric felt light-headed and weak but tried to remain stoic. For Rene, the living nightmare continued. Even though both parents knew beforehand what the diagnosis was likely to be, there is no easy way to hear that your precious infant son has a malignant tumor in the center of his brain. I sat with them for a few minutes while they processed the news. Kedric would tell me later that he was doing everything he could to harvest hope. Blakey had come through the surgery okay, and they were going to help him fight this cruel disease. Rene would tell me how she felt despondent and heartbroken but needed to rally herself to help Blakey get through the next stage of treatment. She felt as if she'd reached her limit. She said, "For a parent, it's really tough to see your child sick. But to see your child sick with cancer, that's unbearable. There's nothing worse than knowing that your kid has a terrible incurable disease." She hoped for a miracle.

The final pathology, with genomic profiling, found a mutation in *RB1* (retinoblastoma 1), a tumor suppressor gene. The final diagnosis was an *RB1* mutated pineoblastoma. The diagnosis was confirmed by methylation-based profiling performed at the National Cancer Institute. This was a bit confusing because pineoblastoma is a malignant tumor usually found in the pineal gland, and Blakey's tumor was situated in the suprasellar region, just above the pituitary gland, nowhere near the pineal gland.

That is a rare tumor in a rare location. The pineal gland (Latin: *pinea*, "pine cone") is a small endocrine organ about the size of a pea that sits at the back end of the third ventricle and secretes melatonin, which has a role in modulation of the circadian rhythm, the wake sleep cycle. Further, the *RB1*, or retinoblastoma gene, refers to the layer of photoreceptors in the retina, at the back of the eye.

There actually is a connection between the pineal gland of the brain and the retina of the eye. Historically, the pineal gland has been referred to as the "third eye" based on its secretion of melatonin in response to light and darkness. In fact, in the 1600s, the pineal gland was considered to be the seat of the soul by the French philosopher, Rene Descartes. But for those of us in neurosurgery, the pineal gland is the site of a variety of tumors that are difficult to reach and tricky to treat. The pathology of the malignant tumor, pineoblastoma, is closely related to the malignant tumor of the eye, retinoblastoma. In fact, the trilateral retinoblastoma is a rare malignant neoplasm affecting children with both intra-ocular retinoblastoma and intracranial pineoblastoma.

But why do we call Blakey's suprasellar tumor a pineoblastoma when it doesn't arise from the pineal gland? The answer has to do with the current reclassification of brain tumors by the WHO, using a hybrid system that includes the standard histologic light-microscope-based diagnosis, pineoblastma, along with the novel molecular signature, in this case, the *RB1* mutation. So, with this new classification scheme, rarely a pineoblastoma can occur in a site remote from the pineal gland. Blakey's tumor is an example of this extremely rare malignant tumor.

The hope is to use molecular profiling someday to develop novel targeted therapies. But currently, we have made more progress in identifying the molecular signatures of brain tumors than developing novel treatments to target these molecular aberrations. Unfortunately, at this time, there is no proven effective targeted therapy for the aggressive *RB1*-mutated pineoblastoma.

Overall, Blakey had a smooth post-op course. He developed some new transient right periorbital swelling immediately after surgery, related to swelling of his scalp from the surgery. This resolved spontaneously after a few days. He was discharged home doing well on New Year's Eve.

Meanwhile, Dr. Jeff Rubens and the medical oncology team were planning his adjuvant therapy, the helper treatment after surgery to keep his cancer in check. For a pineoblastoma, the most effective adjuvant therapy is radiation, which is toxic to the rapidly dividing cancer cells. But we didn't want to use radiation because Blakey was so young. Radiation therapy can cause significant injury to the normal brain, particularly the immature rapidly growing brain of an infant. Deleterious effects of radiation include the development of second tumors over time, cognitive, psychosocial, and endocrine issues, vascular disorders, alopecia, and multiple other problems. Radiation would not be a safe option for Blakey.

We discussed Blakey's case in our tumor board conference and spoke to colleagues around the country to help select the most effective, least toxic regimen of chemotherapy. The oncologists opted to treat with a regimen of intensive chemotherapy called Head Start IV. The regimen began with multi-agent induction chemotherapy consisting of vincristine, cisplatin, etoposide, cyclophosphamide, and methotrexate. The chemotherapy would be followed by tandem autologous bone marrow transplants. The reason for this is that the highly toxic chemotherapy that kills the tumor cells will also destroy normal cells in the patient's bone marrow. The technique involves removing the healthy bone marrow stem cells before further toxic chemotherapy and then replacing them after the treatment.

So, on January 13, Dr. Dan Rhee of general pediatric surgery inserted a Hickman catheter into Blakey's right internal jugular vein that could be repetitively accessed percutaneously (through the skin) to administer the chemotherapy. The chemotherapy regimen began the following day.

A few days after the first round of chemotherapy was completed, Blakey developed a life-threatening complication. On January 22, Rene noted that he appeared ashen and was moaning and abnormally sleepy. His face looked puffy, and his lips and skin appeared dark. Even though he was still recovering from his recent chemotherapy, Rene felt that something was different. It was a mother's intuition. It was about 7 p.m., and there was a change of shift about to happen.

Rene reported her findings to the nurse, who found that Blakey was tachycardic (rapid heart rate) and hypoxic (low oxygen level). A chest X-ray showed cardiomegaly (enlarged heart), and an EKG showed low voltage heart activity. An echocardiogram (sonar study) showed a large pericardial effusion, an excess of fluid within the pericardium (heart sac). The fluid compressed the heart causing cardiac tamponade, preventing it from beating normally and reducing cardiac output causing shock. Blakey became hypotensive (low blood pressure) and was rushed from his room on the floor to the PICU.

In the PICU, an emergency pericardiocentesis was performed at the bedside, in which a cardiologist inserted a needle through the chest wall to aspirate the fluid accumulating around the heart. Eighty milliliters of straw-colored fluid were aspirated from the heart sac. But during the pericardiocentesis, Blakey became bradycardic (low heart rate) and then went into cardiac arrest. His heart had stopped beating. Cardiopulmonary resuscitation was initiated immediately with chest compressions.

One of the doctors came out and told Rene and Kedric that Blakey's heart had stopped and the team was trying to resuscitate him. Kedric went into prayer mode. Rene heard another loud alarm go off. A Code was being called for PICU Bed 27. That was Blakey's room. Rene panicked and rushed back to the PICU on her own and stood outside Blakey's room, where she saw a large crowd of people around her son trying to resuscitate him. The scene was terrifying. Blakey's blood was on the floor and on the gowns of the doctors resuscitating him. Rene could barely stand.

Eric Jelin of general pediatric surgery entered the room and placed Blakey emergently on extracorporeal membranous oxygen (ECMO). ECMO is a life-support system in which blood is pumped into a machine outside the body where carbon dioxide is removed. The blood is then rewarmed, oxygenated, and returned to the body. This gives the heart and lungs a chance to rest. Patients who sustain a cardiac arrest and require ECMO are the sickest of the sick. Many do not survive, and those who survive are often significantly impaired.

Remarkably, little Blakey survived. He was taken off ECMO four days later and transferred out of the PICU two days after that. He recovered rapidly. Miraculously, the old Blakey was back.

Just as Blakey got out of the PICU and things started to settle down, Rene got a call from her sister that their father had become suddenly unresponsive and had suffered a major stroke. It was a living nightmare. Rene rushed to the hospital in Fairfax, Virginia, to be at his side. She was physically and emotionally overwhelmed and wanted to be in two places at the same time. When she arrived in Fairfax, her father deteriorated rapidly, and the doctors told her there was nothing more they could do. He died the next day.

Our hearts went out to Rene. Every time she got a flicker of hope, she was confronted with another disaster. She was incredibly strong, as was her husband. And her son. Blakey continued to make an amazing recovery and was discharged home.

Blakey came back to the hospital for a second round of induction chemotherapy. This time, though, the oncologists reduced the dosages of his chemotherapy regimen. And they eliminated methotrexate, believing that was the most likely culprit responsible for his pericardial tamponade and cardiac arrest. He handled the therapy okay, but the oncologists were unable to harvest enough stem cells to be able to continue with his induction chemotherapy.

Given the severe toxicity from the high-powered Head Start induction chemotherapy regimen, we opted to change plans. We transitioned Blakey to metronomic chemotherapy to maintain his remission while minimizing drug toxicities until a later date when he could tolerate re-intensification chemotherapy and, ultimately, radiation. Metronomic therapy consists of repetitive cycles of low-dose oral chemotherapy along with monthly intrathecal chemotherapy (injected directly into the nervous system by a spinal tap).

As a reporter for CNN, Rene was well-connected and had turned to her colleague, Dr. Sanjay Gupta, CNN's chief medical correspondent, for advice. Dr. Gupta is also a neurosurgeon who did his residency training at the University of Michigan. He serves as an associate chief of neurosurgery at the Grady Memorial Hospital in Atlanta, Georgia, and an associate professor of neurosurgery at the Emory University School of Medicine. He was incredibly helpful to us and generous with his time. He and I spoke frequently during Blakey's hospitalizations, and he provided invaluable advice and support. He helped connect our team with leading oncologists in the United States and around the world.

After two cycles of induction chemotherapy, Blakey's brain MRI was clean, with no evidence of tumor. He had achieved a complete remission. And his left esotropia, the finding that brought him to medical attention, had resolved.

Blakey was a tough little kid and tolerated nine twenty-one-day cycles of this metronomic therapy with only intermittent nausea and bouts of neutropenia (low white blood cell count). He loved being at home with his parents, humming Bob Marley songs and classical music, particularly Mozart's "Serenade #13." And he always loved trying, unsuccessfully, to snap his fingers. He particularly enjoyed cruising the neighborhood in his drop-top electric car. Still, being on all these chemotherapy drugs and traipsing back and forth to the hospital over these months was no walk in the park for Blakey or his parents. But throughout this period his surveillance MRIs continued to show a complete response, with no evidence of residual tumor.

On November 20, 2020, Blakey came to the hospital for his final dose of lumbar intrathecal chemotherapy, which he tolerated well. Blakey completed his last round of metronomic therapy and rang the bell in the oncology clinic, a ritual to celebrate the end of the long ordeal. He went for a final MRI to confirm the continued complete response to therapy and the absence of tumor. The plan was to transition to re-intensification chemotherapy to maintain his complete response and enable him to get a little older at which time he could receive radiation therapy.

We were in the midst of the COVID-19 pandemic and the Children's Hospital had limited visitors to only one person per patient. That meant that while Rene stayed inside with Blakey, poor Kedric had to sit outside in the car the entire time. Things were even more austere on the adult service in the hospital—concern about spread of the virus was so great that no visitors were allowed whatsoever. There were patients who were deathly ill in the ICU, and no family members or friends could be at their side. It was an awful time for patients, families, and health-care providers.

I had been through a lot with Rene and Kedric and kept them abreast of what was happening with the MRI. It was late in the day, and the non-contrast MRI had been completed. I had a look at the scan and saw Rene to let her know that it looked good. We called Kedric on the phone to give him the good news. So far, so good. Then I went to the MRI control room to have a look at the MR images performed after the administration of intravenous gadolinium contrast. I felt a pit in my stomach. It was as if I'd been hit by a ton of bricks.

The tumor had come back with a vengeance. There was diffuse leptomeningeal spread, that is, the tumor had now mushroomed extensively over the surface of the brain and spinal cord, like a poorly applied coating of paint. And there were distant solid tumor metastases in the brain as well. How could this have happened? Blakey had been doing so well, and he had maintained a complete response for months. We all knew that this was a particularly lethal tumor from the get-go, but all the evidence showed that we had the tumor in check.

How could I break the news to Rene and Kedric? They had been through the most miserable year of their lives, and they were emotionally and physically exhausted. It appeared that we were approaching the end of a long dark tunnel, and now this. Even worse, I had already shared with them that the non-contrast scan was clean and that we were just waiting to complete the scan and confirm what we expected—that the tumor was no longer present. We were just waiting to dot the i's and cross the t's.

I had made a rookie mistake. Wanting to keep their spirits high, I gave Rene and Kedric the good news about the clean non-contrast MRI. I should have waited for the entire MRI to be completed before talking to them. Breaking bad news is never a pleasant job. But bad news is much harder to swallow once you have been given a glimpse of hope that is erroneous. I had meant well, but the hope I gave them, the hope I shared, was false hope. I wish I had waited.

I met with Rene and Kedric and broke the news to them. Because of the nature of the circumstances, the hospital made an exception to the rule and allowed Kedric to come back inside to be with his wife and child. It was a somber conversation. I wondered how these two young parents could handle so many setbacks in their long journey with this horrible disease. But they remained strong for their son. And in spite of the findings on his MRI, Blakey awakened from the anesthetic for the study and was in good spirits. They went home and made plans with Dr. Rubens and our oncology team to return for salvage chemotherapy.

The salvage therapy was a regimen called ICE and consisted of three powerful drugs—ifosfamide, carboplatin, and etoposide. The treatment was complicated by seizures, presumably related to neurotoxicity from ifosfamide, so that agent was discontinued and replaced by cyclophosphamide, in a regimen called CCE. Blakey tolerated several cycles of CCE, and miraculously, his MRI showed a second complete response.

The oncologists planned to administer further intensification chemotherapy along with stem cell rescue from an autologous bone marrow transplant, but not enough cells could be mobilized because of the heavy chemotherapy pre-treatment. Blakey began to deteriorate rapidly, with irritability, vomiting, and unsteadiness. There was extensive, overwhelming, diffuse return of his cancer on MRI. He died in the hospital with his family by his side at 3 p.m. on April 14, 2021, eighteen months from the time of his diagnosis and just one month after his second birthday.

In the brief twenty-five months that courageous little Blake Payne lived on this planet, he was destined to spend both birthdays and both Christmases in the hospital. But during that time, he touched many lives. He was a ray of sunshine to his parents, filling their world with happiness and laughter. And he was adored by the medical, surgical, and nursing staff who cared for him at Johns Hopkins.

Throughout the entire ordeal, Rene hung on to hope. She was grateful for the extra year she got to spend with her son when he came off life support. She stressed the value of having hope, even if you don't win the battle in the end. She found solace by tapping into the reservoir of hope. Without hope, Rene felt she would not have been able to keep going on. Even on the last day of Blakey's life, Rene continued to hope for a miracle. Sadly, it didn't come.

Rene wrote a heartbreaking tribute to her late son:

> You taught me how much strength I had stored up in reserve that I didn't know I had. You taught me endurance. You taught me a depth of love I have never experienced. You inspired me to keep going when I wanted to give up. You helped me prioritize what is truly important in this life. I am forever changed because of you, my son. I feel blessed and honored to have been your mom. I wish we had more time together but I'm grateful for the time we had. I am dedicated to fighting pediatric cancer for the rest of my life. I will do it not just to spare other parents from this unbearable pain but I will do it to forever honor you Blake. Your life was not in vain my sweet angel.

After Blakey died, our team from Johns Hopkins and the experts from the US and Canada met in a Zoom symposium in an attempt to develop strategies to improve the outcome and mitigate the life-threatening treatment-related toxicities for the tumor we had all battled with. Suggestions included attempting low-dose conformal proton beam radiation even though he was so young, trying immunotherapy, and exploring novel agents to target other vulnerable molecular pathways expressed by the RB pineoblastoma. The results of the seminar were published in an open-access article in *Neuro-Oncology Advances*, the journal of the Society for Neuro-Oncology.

Rene and Kedric continue to fight passionately against the disease that robbed them of their son. Working with the Pediatric Brain Tumor Foundation, they established the Blake Vince Payne Star Fund to support pineoblastoma research. They were frustrated that of the billions of federal dollars allocated for cancer research, only 4 percent goes to support research in pediatric cancer. One reason for this is the rarity of many types of pediatric cancer. Adult cancers are more common. And Blakey's cancer, an RB1 pineoblastoma that developed in a site remote from the pineal region, is the rarest of the rare.

But that doesn't mean it should be ignored. Research to decipher the molecular signatures of brain tumors can lead to the development of targeted therapies in the form of personalized medicine. These techniques can be applied across the board to develop treatment strategies for multiple tumor types, those that are common and those that are rare. Some cancers that were once considered death sentences are now treatable and curable. When I was in training, acute lymphoblastic leukemia (ALL) was a death sentence, the leading cause of cancer death in children. Today, on the basis of advances in diagnosis and treatment, the majority of children with ALL can be cured. Pediatric brain tumors now lead the list as the number-one cause of cancer death in children.

Unfortunately, firearms are the number-one overall cause of death in children in the United States, and the death rate from firearms in the US has been rising. In contrast, firearms rank no higher than fifth as a cause of childhood mortality in eleven other large, wealthy, industrialized countries.

Inspired by the fighting spirit of her late son, Rene chose to write a children's book in his memory. The idea came to her when she sat by Blakey's side and read to him during his many days in the hospital. He loved books, and he loved having Rene read to him every day. She wrote the book by tapping the words into her iPhone as she sat beside her son in the hospital. She called it *The Miracle Workers: Boy vs. Beast*. The boy's name was Blake. The beast was cancer.

It is an inspirational story about bravery and hope and Blake's adventures in a magical land: "The Miracle Workers will solve every worry. Call on them now and they'll come in a hurry." One hundred percent of the profits from the sale of the book have been donated to support pediatric brain cancer research. The lethal pineoblastoma had stolen the role of motherhood from Rene. *The Miracle Workers* was her way to continue to honor her sweet angel and his life—and to give hope to others.

CHAPTER 10

Judgment

"The general who wins a battle makes many calculations in his temple before the battle is fought. The general who loses makes but few calculations beforehand."

Sun Tzu
Chinese Military General, Philosopher
The Art of War
5th century BC

I was working in my office at Johns Hopkins in the early evening of Thursday, July 29, 2021, preparing a lecture for the medical students, when I got a call from my friend and colleague, Justin Caplan, a cerebrovascular neurosurgeon in my department. It had been a long day, and I was tired. The weather was terrible, with severe storms in the Baltimore area. A tornado had touched down in nearby Columbia, Maryland, and I was waiting for things to clear up a bit before leaving for home.

We were in the midst of the COVID-19 pandemic at the time. Johns Hopkins Hospital was still reeling from its effects and had instituted dramatic alterations in the way we practiced medicine. The number of people infected with the virus nationwide that July had more than quadrupled, with thirteen thousand daily cases at the start of the month, rising to fifty-six thousand at the end of the month.

Dr. Anthony Fauci, director of the National Institute of Allergy and Infectious Diseases and chief medical adviser to the president, was predicting that future COVID-19 surges would be more likely to occur in US cities where the vaccination level was low. Meanwhile, the same day, Fox News host Tucker Carlson accused Fauci of being "the guy who created COVID." I was feeling uneasy about the politicization of the COVID-19 pandemic and felt particularly bad for Fauci, who had dedicated his academic life to the prevention and treatment of multiple infectious diseases, including HIV/AIDS, tuberculosis, Zika, and Ebola. He was a graduate of Cornell Medical School almost a decade before me, and I was blown away by his brilliance when I was a student in the audience hearing him speak.

My colleague Justin got to the point quickly on the phone. "Al, a neurosurgeon friend of mine in North Carolina just called me. He's got a kid in the emergency room with a headache and a large brain tumor. The family wants to come to Hopkins for treatment right away. Can you call them?" He gave me the dad's cell number, and I gave him a call. It was 7:30 p.m.

The dad was Jeff Lehrfeld, and the patient was his seventeen-year-old son, Owen. The family had been spending the week vacationing at the beach in a rental home on Oak Island. Owen had been waking up each morning with progressively worsening headaches, and this time, the headache was followed by copious vomiting. The neurosurgeon who saw Owen in the emergency room ordered a CT scan, which showed a brain tumor in the cerebellum (Latin for "little brain"), the balance center of the brain in the posterior fossa of the skull that regulates motor function.

The medical team in North Carolina felt the tumor was a pilocytic astrocytoma, the most common childhood brain tumor, which arises from the star-shaped supporting astrocytes of the brain. The tumor was causing dangerous compression on the brainstem, the command central portion of the brain. Owen would need urgent surgery. The local team offered to do the operation there, but the family wanted to come to Hopkins. They sent us a digitized copy of the CT scan, and we agreed to accept Owen in transfer.

The transfer was easier said than done. Jeff and his wife, Kim, loaded up their cars and hit the road that night to bring Owen to see us at Johns Hopkins. Owen rode with Jeff, and his monozygotic (identical) twin brother Tyler rode separately with Kim. The trip was not fun for Owen, who had to make frequent stops to throw up in gas stations and convenience stores and parking lots. They arrived at their home in Fulton, Maryland, a suburb of Baltimore, sometime after 3 a.m. Fulton is a charming, vibrant town in Howard County, considered one of the nicest places to live in Maryland.

After their unpleasant journey from North Carolina, Jeff, Kim, and Owen made the thirty-minute trip to Johns Hopkins, where I met them in the emergency room early Friday morning. Owen was still having dry heaves. I helped them get admitted to the ER, where we gave Owen some intravenous fluids for hydration. We also administered intravenous dexamethasone, a steroid, to reduce the intracranial pressure from the edema caused by his tumor. Then I sat down and spoke to Owen and his parents.

Owen was a previously healthy seventeen-year-old boy who was an honor student in high school about to begin his senior year in two weeks. He was also an athlete on the track team. The first time he noted a problem was two months earlier in a track meet when he felt he was losing his balance and felt a bit unsteady on his feet. The balance problem continued, and the next thing he noticed was that his racing speed got worse. Specifically, he found that his clock time on the four-hundred-meter dash, his choice race, had fallen by 1.5 seconds. Over the next few weeks, he began to feel more unsteady when he was walking, and he noted some difficulty with eye-hand coordination that he'd never experienced before. He saw his primary care physician, who thought it might be an inner ear problem and prescribed Zyrtec, an antihistamine, and salt. His doctor set up an appointment for Owen to see an ear, nose, and throat specialist in a few weeks. But the balance problem persisted and got worse.

About one month before I met him, Owen started experiencing headaches. They were often present in the morning when he awakened, and they were usually located at the back of his head. They tended to be short in duration, lasting several minutes, but over time, they increased in frequency and severity. They often occurred when he changed position, particularly in the morning when he got out of bed and stood up. But sometimes, they came on later in the day when he arose from sitting in a chair.

There are multiple causes of headache in children, and most of them are not something to get overly concerned about. But morning headaches catch the attention of the neurologist and neurosurgeon, as they may sometimes, but certainly not always, be associated with an intracranial space-occupying lesion, such as a brain tumor.

There are several reasons for this. When we sleep, our bodies are generally flat or close to it, which means the venous drainage of the brain is not as robust as it is when we are upright and subject to the effects of gravity. Thus, in the presence of a brain tumor, the recumbent position of sleep can contribute to increasing the intracranial pressure with resultant exacerbation of headaches. Sleep can exacerbate a brain tumor headache in another way. During sleep, we tend to hypoventilate, breathing a little slower. This tends to allow carbon dioxide to accumulate in the blood vessels. Carbon dioxide is a potent arterial vasodilator and can increase blood flow to the brain. In the presence of a tumor in the brain, this excess blood flow can further increase the intracranial pressure, leading to a worsening of headaches.

By the time Owen went on vacation with his family to Oak Island, the headaches were coming on every morning. His balance problem became more obvious while he was on vacation. He was active physically and saw that his eye-hand coordination was off when he was playing touch football on the beach. His swimming didn't feel right. He knew something was wrong but didn't know what it was.

On Thursday morning, July 29, 2001, the fifth day of his vacation, he awakened and sat down at his computer to do a Python programming module as part of a Johns Hopkins University Applied Physics Lab he was taking as a high school student. He began to feel unwell and then developed a sudden, severe headache followed by profuse vomiting. At that point, Owen's parents promptly brought him to the emergency room at Wilmington Hospital in North Carolina, where again the cause of the problem wasn't immediately clear. The CT scan showed the surprise finding of a cerebellar brain tumor that prompted his transfer to us at Johns Hopkins.

After taking the history, I examined Owen and found him to be extremely bright but somewhat pale from his repetitive bouts of emesis and sleep deprivation. There was a six-centimeter maculopapular patch (an area of flat and raised hyperpigmentation) on the skin over his left abdomen. There was another pigmented tan patch on his right upper arm. His eye exam was normal except for a two-millimeter dark-brown macule (small, flat dark spot) at about six o'clock on his left iris. His visual acuity was perfect, and his retinal exam was normal, with flat optic disks, subsequently confirmed on a formal dilated eye exam by ophthalmology. The only other remarkable physical finding was truncal ataxia, with Owen veering a little to the right when he tried to do tandem heel-to-toe walking, indicative of difficulty with his balance related to the tumor in his cerebellum.

Owen threw up twice in our emergency room but began to feel a little better with the IV hydration and steroids. It was uncomfortable for him to lie flat on his back for the duration of the MRI of his brain and spine. The study was performed without and with the administration of intravenous contrast, and it gave us a clearer picture of the anatomy and geometry of the posterior fossa mass.

There was a large cystic mass, measuring five centimeters in diameter, filling the upper part of the cerebellum, along with an adjacent smaller enhancing mural nodule. This was the solid portion of the tumor, measuring 1.5 centimeters in diameter, sitting at the very top of the cerebellum, just beneath the tentorium, the fibrous roof at the top of the cerebellum. There was edema surrounding the tumor, causing pressure on the brainstem. The cerebellar tonsils, the lower portion of the cerebellum, were being squeezed inferiorly such that they were herniated through the foramen magnum, the opening at the base of the skull, compressing the spinal cord. The tumor was obstructing the ventricular system, causing hydrocephalus (water on the brain) with enlargement of the lateral and third ventricles and increased pressure in the head.

The MRI of the spine was normal. Incidental note was made of a small shadow in the right lobe of the liver, felt likely to be a benign cyst.

Our neuroradiologists read the MRI and the CT scan from the outside hospital. The tumor appeared to be a pilocytic astrocytoma, a benign tumor, considered by the World Health Organization (WHO) to be grade 1, the most favorable grade possible. The pilocytic astrocytoma is a well-circumscribed tumor that was first described in 1931 by Harvey Cushing but called a spongioblastoma at that time. The most common location for a pilocytic astrocytoma in a child is the cerebellum.

Owen's tumor was large and causing significant brain compression. It was clear that surgery would be needed, both to confirm the diagnosis and take pressure off the brain. The standard surgical approach would be a posterior fossa craniotomy with the patient positioned prone (face down). A portion of the base of the skull is temporarily removed (and later replaced), and the surgeon works from below, going through the fluid-filled cyst up to the top of the cerebellum to finally excise the solid portion of the tumor. It's a straightforward procedure and one of the standard operations we do in pediatric neurosurgery.

But there was something unusual about Owen's case, and we didn't realize it until after we had taken a careful look at the MRI for surgical planning. On the T2-weighted MRI sequences, one of the standard MRI pulse sequences based on magnetic relaxation time, we saw several dark spots inside the otherwise bright portion of the solid tumor. We wondered if they might represent blood vessels. If so, that would be distinctly unusual for a pilocytic astrocytoma. It could mean that the lesion was a vascular tumor, one filled with blood vessels. One such tumor, the hemangioblastoma, can also be cystic and solid, just like Owen's tumor, and can occur in the cerebellum in children and even mimic the pilocytic astrocytoma. Hemangioblastomas are benign, highly vascular, and very rare tumors, accounting for about 1–2 percent of all brain tumors. They are even more uncommon in children.

Owen's laboratory values all came back normal, except that he had polycythemia (too many red blood cells), the opposite of anemia. His hemoglobin was elevated at 17.4 grams per deciliter. It was noteworthy that Owen's mother, Kim, also had polycythemia that required phlebotomy (bloodletting) in the past. Polycythemia can have many causes, but the brain tumor most associated with polycythemia is the hypervascular hemangioblastoma. That tumor causes polycythemia by secreting the glycoprotein erythropoietin, which stimulates the production of red blood cells. So, this was another piece of information that led us to believe that Owen's tumor might more likely be a hemangioblastoma than a pilocytic astrocytoma.

For the casual reader, it might seem to be just an academic exercise in trying to distinguish a hemangioblastoma from a pilocytic astrocytoma, like splitting hairs. They are both benign tumors, and when they cause symptoms from mass effect, they both need to be removed. But for the surgeon planning the operative approach, this distinction is of paramount importance. If Owen's tumor were a hemangioblastoma and we chose to use the conventional trajectory for removing a pilocytic astrocytoma, working from below, going through the cyst, and attacking the bottom of the solid tumor first, we could potentially cause torrential bleeding and even exsanguinate the patient. That's because the hemangioblastoma is a hornet's nest. It's a hypervascular tumor, a tangle of blood vessels, receiving its blood supply from the superior cerebellar arteries situated on top of the tumor, on the "dark side of the moon" so to speak. The proper way to remove a hypervascular tumor like a hemangioblastoma is to interrupt its blood supply early, in this case, coming at the tumor from above rather than from below.

So, we asked my neurosurgical colleague, Dr. Fernando Gonzalez, to perform a cerebral angiogram, specialized imaging of the blood vessels. With Owen sedated, Dr. Gonzalez passed a soft catheter through the common femoral artery in the leg and threaded it up to the blood vessels of the brain under fluoroscopic guidance. Next, he injected contrast material into the blood vessels while taking X-rays of the head. And lo and behold, the tumor was indeed a hemangioblastoma.

It was hypervascular, fed by branches of the right superior cerebellar artery, with drainage from the tumor going deep in the midline into the great vein of Galen. Dr. Gonzalez attempted to embolize the tumor, hoping to close off some of the blood supply by injecting glue into the vessels supplying it, to help make our planned surgical resection safer. But the blood vessels supplying the tumor were so tortuous (winding) that it wasn't possible to advance the microcatheter close enough to the tumor to perform the embolization.

Owen had been admitted to the pediatric intensive care unit and returned there after the angiogram. He was feeling much better once the IV fluids and steroids had kicked in. I sat down with Owen and his parents to go over plans and obtain informed consent for the surgery. It was clear to me that this was a high-functioning, very bright family, and Jeff and Kim were appropriately terrified. As is sometimes the case, the child helps the parents through a serious health crisis. That's exactly what happened here. Owen was the calmest of the three of them. He had known for a couple of months that there was something very wrong with him. He was relieved that we had found an answer and had developed a plan to deal with it.

Jeff had a strong medical background, serving as the chief financial officer of the Priority Partners Managed Care Organization, which provides health-care insurance for over 340,000 Maryland residents. Kim was a risk management analyst for the US Food and Drug Administration. They were both medically savvy and had a lot of questions. I showed them the scans and the angiogram and outlined our plan of attack. Kim would later tell me that she was scared out of her wits and remembered everything that day as a blur. While Jeff signed the consent, Owen was texting his friends to keep them up to date with plans.

We performed the surgery on the following day, Wednesday, August 4, 2021. I worked with Risheng Xu, an MD, PhD, senior neurosurgery resident. Risheng is one of the most talented surgeons I have ever met. There's a video of him on YouTube when he was only fifteen years old, in which he gave a virtuoso classical piano recital at a Houston Young Artists Performance. He is a virtuoso neurosurgeon as well.

Owen was anesthetized and placed prone in a Concorde position. The Concorde position mimics the tailless supersonic jet, which has a narrow fuselage and a forward "beak" that is turned slightly down. By elevating Owen's head slightly, we were able to stand behind him and work in the narrow space above the cerebellum to close off the blood supply to the tumor early in order to make the resection safer, using gravity to help retract the cerebellum downward. Once we opened the skull and exposed the cerebellum, we used magnetic resonance image guidance and ultrasonography to insert a thin, flexible catheter into the tumor cyst to decompress it and give us more working room at the top of the tumor in order to pick off the blood supply.

We worked under the guidance of the operating microscope and coagulated and cut off the numerous arterial feeders one by one in a long, tedious procedure. Since we had good exposure at the top of the tumor, we were able to identify the venous drainage early on and protect it until after we took the incoming blood supply. That's a general principle of surgery for this kind of tumor. If we were to interrupt the venous drainage of a vascular tumor before cutting off the arterial blood supply, we could encounter a situation of explosive hemorrhage—the blood getting into the tumor wouldn't be able to get out.

The surgery was long. It lasted seven and a half hours, but we were happy that we were able to get the entire tumor out without any misadventures. The frozen section came back as we were operating and was indeed a hemangioblastoma, which was no surprise. The final pathology returned the following week, after all the special stains were done, and confirmed the diagnosis. Microscopic examination showed polygonal cells with hyperchromatic (darkly staining) nuclei and vacuolar (containing small fluid cavities) cytoplasm. It was a classic hemangioblastoma.

I met with Jeff and Kim in the waiting room and gave them the good news. It was an emotional encounter, as it always is, and tears flowed. Jeff and Kim were fortunate to have Jeff's colleague and friend, Dr. Kayode Williams, the chief medical officer at Priority Partners, stay by their side in the waiting room and throughout Owen's hospitalization. He helped usher them through a very scary period in their lives.

We went to see Owen in the intensive care unit and gave him the good news that we got the tumor out and that it was benign. He was far less emotional than his parents and seemed unfazed. He told me later that he took things in stride because he went into surgery knowing that everything was going to be okay. Owen continued to make a nice recovery and was eating breakfast the next morning and was up walking around.

But we weren't done yet.

The hemangioblastoma is a rare, histologically benign, WHO grade 1 vascular tumor. As I noted, hemangioblastomas are particularly rare in children. The mean age of onset of solitary sporadic hemangioblastomas is fifty years. But there is an uncommon though serious disorder called von Hippel-Lindau (VHL) disease, in which hemangioblastomas occur in younger patients, along with other benign and malignant tumors of the central nervous system and other parts of the body. The mean age of onset of hemangioblastomas in VHL is twenty-five years, much closer to Owen's age. So, we had concerns about Owen and felt he should be screened for VHL.

VHL is a rare inherited disorder with an incidence of one in thirty-six thousand individuals. It is caused by a single mutation of the VHL tumor suppressor gene on chromosome 3. The neurosurgical hallmarks of VHL are hemangiomas of the brain and spinal cord. But there are many tumors elsewhere in the body as well. VHL patients can develop retinal angiomas that can lead to blindness. They can also have cysts in the kidneys and pancreas, and tumors of the adrenal glands called pheochromocytomas that can secrete hormones that may cause dangerous elevations in blood pressure. There can be other noncancerous tumors of the inner ear, liver, and lungs. One of the most feared complications for patients with VHL is the development of clear cell carcinoma of the kidney (kidney cancer), which has become the number-one cause of death in patients with VHL.

It is also noteworthy that patients with VHL can develop polycythemia, which Owen and his mother had, as a result of secretion of erythropoietin from their hemangioblastomas. However, the presence of polycythemia is not a diagnostic criterion for VHL, as patients with solitary hemangioblastomas can have polycythemia for the same reason—erythropoietin secretion by the tumor.

VHL is a dangerous inherited cancer predisposing disorder, which we know much more about in recent years, thanks to advances in clinical genetics. The disease was named for two eminent European physicians, Eugen von Hippel and Arvid Lindau.

Von Hippel was a German ophthalmologist who was born in Konigsberg, Germany (now Kaliningrad, Russia), in 1867, two years after the end of the Civil War in the US. He described the retinal angiomas of the disorder in 1904. Arvid Lindau was born in Malmö, Sweden, to a military family in 1892. He earned an MD and a PhD and became a pathologist and bacteriologist. He was awarded a Rockefeller Fellowship, which allowed him to spend time working in the laboratory of Harvey Cushing in Boston. The two developed a close collaboration and became good friends. Lindau described the cerebellar hemangioblastomas in VHL. He was the person who linked the ocular, cerebral, and visceral components into a single disorder in 1926.

Our excitement about how well Owen was doing was mitigated by the concern that he could actually have VHL. The concern was not only for Owen, but also for his identical twin brother, Tyler. This introduced a significant amount of anxiety, primarily felt by Jeff and Kim, along with most of Owen's physicians. Curiously, Owen and Tyler were cool and calm throughout the ordeal. I still don't know how they managed to have so much self-control. We engaged a multidisciplinary team at Hopkins and did an elaborate workup with a series of scans and lab tests. Ultimately, the genetic testing proved negative. Owen did not have VHL. We were all elated by the news.

Somewhat ironically, Kim's colleagues at the FDA were involved in the recent approval of a new drug, belzutifan, a hypoxia inducible factor inhibitor, for treating adults with VHL-associated tumors, particularly renal cell cancer. Fortunately, her own Owen will not need that drug.

Owen made a remarkable recovery. He was discharged home from the hospital five days after surgery on no medication. He had some neck stiffness that resolved after a few weeks of physical therapy. He was able to begin his senior year of high school on time with all his classmates. During the week of his vacation, just before he was hospitalized for his brain tumor, he learned that he had been chosen for his dream position, to be the drum major of the school's marching band. Two days after he was discharged from the hospital following his tumor resection, he proudly led the band as drum major and sent me a picture of him taken from behind that showed off his midline posterior fossa surgical scar.

Owen finished high school with honors and is now a senior at the University of Maryland in College Park, where he was on the swim team and ran track. He plays pickup basketball to stay active. He is majoring in mechanical engineering with a minor physics and robotics, and a grade point average (GPA) of 3.96. His identical twin brother is majoring in computer science at Johns Hopkins with a minor in computer-integrated surgery and a double major in political science. Owen is a member of the Terps Racing Club in college where students design and build an off-road vehicle and take part in national competitions. Of note, the two brothers each wrote their college entrance essays about the importance of resilience in coping with Owen's brain surgery. Four years after his operation, Owen's MRI shows no evidence of a tumor.

Owen's case highlights the critical role of surgical judgment and surgical planning in patient care. The previous cases in this book have focused on the importance of personal, human non-technical factors as an adjunct to the technical innovations that have given us incredible tools to perform microsurgery. While we're immersed in an era of technology, it's crucial not to forget the role of basic human factors like compassion and empathy in the art of healing. In simple terms, it means remembering to see the patient as a person.

But to effectively carry out surgery, the wise surgeon relies on meticulous planning and surgical judgment. A surgeon may be the kindest person in the world and have access to state-of-the-art equipment, but without thoughtful planning and judgment, the operative results could be catastrophic. One of the most important aspects of any operation is what happens before the patient even enters the OR.

In some ways, a surgeon planning an operation is similar to a general going to battle. I began this chapter with the words of the Chinese military strategist Sun Tzu ("Master Sun") recommending to generals that they spend time preparing in their "temple" before the battle is fought. This is not a new concept. His book, *The Art of War*, was allegedly written on sewn-together slats of bamboo over 2,500 years ago. Its main message is that whenever possible, it is wisest to avoid war with diplomacy. Sun Tzu went on to say this more eloquently, "The supreme art of war is to subdue the enemy without fighting."

There are parallels for the neurosurgeon caring for a child with a brain tumor. Is surgery necessary in the first place? Just because an operation can be done doesn't necessarily mean it should be done. The good surgeon knows when to operate. The great surgeon knows when not to operate. Some tumors may remain stable and can be followed with serial surveillance MRIs, particularly if the risks of making a tissue diagnosis are high. If surgery is necessary, what is the goal? Is it simply to make a diagnosis or to perform a radical resection as well? Some brain tumors, such as the germinoma, a rare malignant tumor arising from primitive cells, don't require radical resection as they are highly responsive to chemotherapy and radiation. If the tumor needs to be removed, what is the least invasive way to remove it? That's where thoughtful preoperative planning comes in. There's an old Hebrew proverb that goes, "The art of surgery is the ability to use superior judgment to avoid having to use superior skills."

Once in the OR, attention is focused on basic surgical technique—careful handling of tissue, meticulous dissection, cutting, sewing, and tying. Even the most complex operations are simply a series of basic maneuvers. Attention to detail is imperative because a single small error can lead to a huge intraoperative complication. The skilled surgeon is not the one who operates the quickest, but rather the one who operates the smoothest. The best surgeon practices economy of movement and is always thinking several steps ahead. There are no unnecessary actions. The surgeon sets the tone in the OR so that the entire team is relaxed and able to perform with maximal efficiency. I like to play music and find that it keeps the staff happy and calm and working together, particularly for long cases.

Astley Paston Cooper (1768–1841), the celebrated British surgeon and anatomist, said, "The best surgeon, like the best general, is he who makes the fewest mistakes." Cooper, by the way, is remembered as an eccentric but ardent vivisectionist who, as a young man, stole his neighbors' pets to perform postmortem dissections. Later in life, he was able to pay others to steal bodies for him, and in the late 1700s, he organized a group of body snatchers in London who supplied him with a large number of corpses. He performed numerous public dissections on executed criminals and lectured his audience about the details of comparative anatomy. Cooper's extensive studies of anatomy enabled him to become a pioneering, though unconventional, surgeon of his era.

The concept of surgical judgment was of supreme importance in Owen's case. When we first planned the surgery, our impression was that we were dealing with a pilocytic astrocytoma. That made good sense at the time. The pilocytic astrocytoma is the most common primary cerebellar brain tumor in children, and we and several neuroradiologists called that the diagnosis after looking at the imaging. It was only after careful analysis of the MRIs that we identified the abnormal tangle of blood vessels that suggested that the tumor was more likely a hemangioblastoma.

The distinction is critical because had we approached the tumor with the standard corridor we use to remove a pilocytic astrocytoma, we would have encountered an angry tangle of blood vessels before we could control the blood supply to the tumor, which could have caused life-threatening bleeding. It's the simple mistakes in planning and executing an operation that can lead to complex problems.

There is great power and beauty in simplicity. Owen's hemangioblastoma resection reminds me that a complex operation is merely the summation of a series of simple maneuvers.

But finding simplicity can be elusive and is not always simple. Nevertheless, the goal of the surgeon should always be to strive to simplify the operation, as it may sometimes be the best way to achieve the optimal outcome.

The importance of simplicity in surgery is illustrated by a story about the pioneer American pediatric surgeon, Robert Edward Gross, who, in 1947, became surgeon-in-chief and Ladd Professor of Children's Surgery at Boston Children's Hospital/ Harvard Medical School. As a young man, Gross was given a copy of Harvey Cushing's two-volume Pulitzer Prize-winning biography of William Osler, which cemented his desire to become a doctor. As a student at Harvard Medical School, Gross recalled the thrill of sitting in the amphitheater to watch Cushing operate. But the thrill was gone when Cushing asked him to identify himself and then embarrassed him by throwing him out of the OR, telling him to return when he became a real doctor.

Gross rose to international recognition when he was chief resident in surgery at Boston Children's Hospital. At that time, he cared for Lorraine Sweeney, a seven-year-old girl from Brighton, Massachusetts, who suffered from extreme fatigue and a constant buzzing in her chest. Workup demonstrated that the problem was a patent ductus arteriosus (PDA), a persistent communication between the aorta and pulmonary artery that had failed to close after birth. At the time, there was no treatment for a PDA, and patients with the disorder usually died at a young age.

Working in the autopsy room and animal lab, Gross had developed a simple operation to ligate (tie off) the PDA, but his boss, William E. Ladd, the Surgeon-in-Chief at Boston Children's, prohibited him from doing it because he felt the procedure was too risky and no one had successfully violated the sanctity of the human heart. So young Gross, not lacking in courage, waited until Ladd was on vacation on a boat in Europe, and on August 26, 1938, he successfully ligated Sweeney's PDA. Ladd returned enraged and promptly fired Gross, but he was forced to rehire him when word got out that Gross had performed the first successful congenital heart surgery in the world. And in 1947, against the wishes of Ladd, Gross followed Ladd and became surgeon-in-chief at Boston Children's Hospital and the inaugural William E. Ladd Professor of Children's Surgery there.

The story provides a fascinating look at the inner dynamics of the origin of congenital heart surgery at one of the premier children's hospitals in the world. Equally fascinating is that Gross was born blind in one eye due to a congenital cataract. Thus, he had only monocular vision and did Sweeney's operation and all of his master surgeries with only one working eye. And throughout his career, none of his colleagues were aware of that.

But the story also demonstrates the power of simplicity in surgery, and how the application of a single suture in the right place can change the world. Gross was well aware of that and famously pronounced, "If an operation is difficult, you are not doing it properly."

In pediatric neurosurgery, the hemangioblastoma is a rare, very treacherous tumor because of its extreme vascularity. While the hemangioblastoma is particularly rare in children, it is the most common primary cerebellar tumor in adults. Over the course of my career, I have operated on several cases of hemangioblastoma, and each one requires meticulous preparation and evokes strong memories.

One of the most remarkable patients I cared for was Frank Kitsis. Frank was a sixty-nine-year-old pharmacist in Belmont, Massachusetts, who noticed that he was veering to the left when he was driving. His wife, June, noticed that as well and was more concerned about it than Frank was. Frank also observed that his golf game was off, and he was slicing the ball more often, usually to the left.

This was back in September 1989, and at the time, I was working at the Tufts New England Medical Center in Boston, having completed ten years of neurosurgery residency training just two years earlier. Frank came to see me, which was somewhat unusual, because I was a pediatric neurosurgeon and served as chief of pediatric neurosurgery at the Floating Hospital for Infants and Children at Tufts. But as a pediatric neurosurgeon, I was also board-certified in general neurosurgery and did care for adult patients as well, so it wasn't all that unusual for him to see me.

His neurological exam was remarkable only for some dysmetria (lack of coordination) on the left side of his body and an ataxic gait (impairment of balance when walking), with him tending to veer to the left. We got an MRI that showed a contrast-enhancing tumor at the top of his cerebellum that looked vascular. A cerebral angiogram confirmed the vascularity of the tumor, which we felt was most likely a hemangioblastoma. It looked very much like Owen's tumor, except it was solid only, with no cyst, and it was on the left side, not the right.

I met with Frank and went over the films and made a plan. The tumor was causing symptoms and should come out. There was something else unusual about Frank, though—he was the father of Rick Kitsis, who was married to my sister Liz. Rick and Liz had been married for four years and had a two-year-old boy named Jeff. At the time, Rick was a cardiology fellow and Liz was a rheumatology fellow at the Albert Einstein College of Medicine in New York City.

Frank asked me to do the surgery and take the tumor out. I told him I didn't think that was a great idea. I had recently completed years of training and was young and somewhat fearless at the time, much more fearless than I am now. But I was not stupid.

"Frank I shouldn't do your surgery" I said. "You are family to me. What happens if I screw something up and have a complication? That would not be good for either of us. I wouldn't be able to live with myself. I don't want that risk. I'd never be able to talk to my sister or Rick again. I'd never be able to go to Thanksgiving dinners with the family. I'm going to refer you to another neurosurgeon in Boston who can do the procedure. He is superb. You'll really like him."

"Don't sweat it Al," Frank said. "You're family, but you're not a blood relative. I have confidence in you. Everything will be okay. I'll see this other guy. But I've already decided I want you to do the case."

I referred him to Robert Ojemann, Professor of Neurosurgery at the Massachusetts General Hospital/Harvard Medical School, and a world renowned brain tumor surgeon. Ojemann was also a very kind man—when I sent patients to him for a second opinion, he would routinely send them back to me, knowing that I was the new guy in town. He didn't have to do that. He was a true gentleman. Frank saw Ojemann, who agreed with my assessment. Ojemann knew it was a complex case and agreed to do the surgery. Frank liked Ojemann a lot. But he came back to see me.

"Al, Ojemann is terrific and I realize he's a worldclass neurosurgeon. But I still want you to do my operation. I'm nervous. I know you. I would feel more comfortable if you did it."

We went back and forth over the next few days, and I declined several times. I remembered the immortal Wilder Penfield's words (see Chapter 17) before he was forced to remove his own sister's brain tumor: "A wise physician will never 'doctor' himself or members of his family if he can help it." He followed his own warning but noted: "And yet there are times that he must act."

Although I would never operate on a blood relative or recommend that anyone do so, there is a precedent for this. William Stewart Halsted of Johns Hopkins, the father of modern surgery, operated on his own mother in 1882 when he was only thirty years old. She was quite ill with gallstones, and he performed a cholecystectomy (gallbladder resection), carrying out the life-saving surgery at 2 a.m. on her own kitchen table. Victor Horsley, ground-breaking surgeon of the National Hospital at Queen Square in London, England, operated unsuccessfully on his own son for epilepsy. That was also in the late 1800s. Those days were long gone, and I stood firm.

But Frank was insistent. He wasn't a blood relative. It would be okay. He was frightened and felt comfortable with me. Ultimately, I got Liz and Rick involved, and they knew the risks, spoke to Frank, and decided that I should go ahead and be Frank's surgeon. So reluctantly, I agreed.

We carried out the operation much the same way as we did for Owen, with the major difference that we did Frank's case with him asleep but bolt upright in the sitting position rather than the stealth position we used for Owen, to take full advantage of gravity retracting the cerebellum downward so we could work on top of it. I'm always a little nervous when I begin a complex case, and this time, I was a little more so than usual because of whose head we were working on.

I always like to keep the mood light in the OR, but I was pretty serious when we began this case and announced to the OR team: "Look, this guy is the father of my sister's husband, so please don't let me mess things up. He needs to do okay, or I'll never be able to face my family again."

The mood was solemn but relaxed. The team got the message, and we were off to a good start. About an hour and a half into the case, I had the head open and was working under the microscope, exposing the tumor, when the anesthesiologist gave me a message that I'd never heard before. "Dr. Cohen, things are going well, but I just want you to know that the patient has not made any urine so far."

That was somewhat unusual, I thought, because we had placed a Foley catheter in his bladder, and he was getting intravenous fluids and should have been making urine. I am usually pretty even-tempered in the OR, but I was clearly upset at the news.

"How could you let something like this happen?" I asked. "You know I'm anxious about the case, and now I've got this guy in the sitting position with the tumor exposed, and I find out that he's made no urine since we started an hour and a half ago? You're killing me. Can someone please go under the drapes and see what's going on?"

I continued operating, trying to keep my cool. The silence was broken ten minutes later when the anesthesiologist spoke again: "Dr. Cohen, I'm sorry. I think we've got a problem. We sent the medical student under the drapes to investigate, and he tried to manipulate the Foley catheter, but in the process, the catheter came out completely. And the balloon that locks it in the bladder is still inflated."

"You've got to be kidding! How could this be happening?" I asked again, trying to remain calm but clearly in a state of disbelief. The Foley catheter has a balloon that we dilate to keep it inside the bladder and prevent it from slipping out. For the Foley to have come out with the balloon still dilated means that someone would have accidentally had to pull the device out with the large balloon traversing the narrow urethra. This would be the cause of intense pain if the patient were awake. And here we were in the midst of a delicate operation without the ability to effectively monitor the patient's fluid status.

After several deep breaths, I calmly asked, "Could someone please go back under the drapes and place a new Foley catheter?"

After one of the longest ten-minute periods I can remember, the anesthesiologist announced, "Dr. Cohen, we were able to get a new Foley catheter in, and he's making good urine, and all vital signs are stable."

Whew. That was music to my ears. It was no easy task to work in darkness under the drapes and place a Foley catheter into a patient's bladder while he was under general anesthesia in the sitting position. We focused on the tumor resection, which was tedious but went well. We were able to resect the vascular tumor, which proved to be a hemangioblastoma. We finished the case after several hours, and Frank awoke nicely, alert, talking, and following commands. A few rocky hours in the OR, but a happy ending.

A lot of time has passed since I removed Frank's tumor in the early stages of my career. Many years have gone by, but I remember the experience vividly. Rick and Liz climbed the academic ladder. Liz is now a professor of rheumatology and the senior associate dean at Albert Einstein, and Rick is a professor of medicine and cell biology with an endowed chair in cerebrovascular research. I am wiser too. From that day forward, I decided never again to operate on a member of the family, even if they were not bound to me by blood. That would be a job for someone else.

On the third day after Frank's surgery, I met up with him while he was going for a walk in the hospital hallway outside his room. He was a tough, unflappable guy but was always in good spirits. "How are you getting along, Frank?" I asked him.

"Overall, I'm doing okay," he said. "Just some pain at the incision site, though it seems to be getting better each day. But I've gotta tell you, Al, I don't understand it. I've never peed this well since I was a teenager!"

Oh my God! I realized immediately what must have happened. Frank likely had some underlying degree of BPH, benign prostatic hyperplasia. This is a common condition in men as they age, in which there is a noncancerous enlargement of the prostate gland that surrounds the urethra, the tube that carries urine from the bladder to the penis. This condition often leads to difficulty emptying the bladder. The episode in the OR when the Foley catheter came out with the balloon still inflated had essentially given Frank the urological procedure called TURP, transurethral resection of the prostate.

So, I told Frank about what happened in the OR. At the time, it was no laughing matter. But with Frank doing well and his discharge home imminent, we both had a good laugh. With a sigh of relief, though, I silently recalled my residency training mantra: Better to be lucky than good.

Struggling to put a positive spin on what had transpired, I turned to him and said, "Frank, you're a fortunate man. Someone up there must be looking out for you. You got two operations for the price of one!"

CHAPTER 11

Borrowed Time

"Optimism doesn't mean that you are blind to the reality of the situation. It means that you remain motivated to seek a solution to whatever problems arise."

Tenzin Gyatso
The Dalai Lama

"There was a bump on top of her head. I could see it, and I could feel it. It was as hard as a rock. I knew something was wrong."

Those were the words of Blessing Ilobi describing the first thing she remembers about the saga that would forever change the life of her beautiful infant daughter, Chizara, as well as the lives of her entire family.

It was the middle of February in 2021, during the height of the COVID-19 pandemic, and Blessing was giving her young six-and-a-half-month-old daughter a bath at their home in Columbia, Maryland. Chizara, nicknamed Zara, had been perfectly healthy. The name Chizara means "god answered my prayers" in Igbo, the language of the ethnic group in southeastern Nigeria, where Blessing grew up. Zara was born at term at 3 a.m. on July 14, 2020, at Howard University Hospital in Washington, DC, via spontaneous vaginal delivery following an uncomplicated pregnancy. Her birth weight was seven pounds, six ounces.

Zara was diagnosed at birth with sickle cell trait, meaning that she had inherited a single copy of the gene that causes sickle cell disease, a disorder in which the red blood cells are abnormally crescent (sickle) shaped, which can cause problems including anemia, infection, stroke, and pain syndromes. Kids with sickle cell trait are carriers and can pass the disease on to their offspring, but don't develop the disease themselves. She had bilateral postaxial polydactyly, meaning that there was an extra finger on the ulnar side of each hand adjacent to the pinky. The extra digits were removed surgically in an uncomplicated procedure when she was a few months old.

Despite the excitement of Zara's birth, times had not been easy for Blessing. Two weeks after Zara's arrival, Blessing's dad passed away in Nigeria. She was unable to attend her father's funeral because it was the height of the COVID-19 pandemic.

Blessing and her husband, Ike, had both grown up in Abuja, Nigeria. Blessing went to college there and studied finance. Ike emigrated to the United States in 2010 after winning a visa lottery. He took a job as a nurse at the Clifton T. Perkins Psychiatric Hospital in Jessup, Maryland. Blessing came to the US in 2016 to visit a cousin in Atlanta, Georgia. She met Ike for the first time at a wedding in New York City, where her cousin was marrying a friend of Ike's who was a theater actor. Blessing was a bridesmaid, and Ike was a groomsman. They dated for six months and married on April 27, 2017. Blessing moved to Maryland with

Ike and took a job as a home health nurse at the Capital City Rehabilitation and Healthcare Center.

Blessing worked as a home health nurse, and when she noticed the bump on Zara's head during the bath, she knew that she was feeling her anterior fontanelle, which was abnormally raised and firm. From personal experience, she knew that was abnormal because she remembered feeling the fontanelle on her three-year-old son Chuka when he was an infant, and it was much softer and usually sunken. Chuka translates as "supreme god" from Igbo. The anterior fontanelle is the soft spot on top of the head in the midline at a region called the bregma, which is the junction of the coronal and sagittal sutures. It is open in infants and usually closes at about a year and a half of life. The anterior fontanelle can be an indicator of what's going on inside the skull. It is usually soft and sunken, but it can be full and even tense when the baby is crying, which is normal. Blessing's concern about her daughter was that the fontanelle was raised and tense even when she wasn't crying.

Over the next few days, Zara became fussy. She slept poorly and spent most nights awake, crying. She seemed to cry more during the night than in the daytime. In the daytime, she often would rest her head on a chair or pillow, as if she were uncomfortable. She became more withdrawn and stopped playing with her brother.

"I noticed that her poop became very hard and looked like small pellets," Blessing recalled. "That didn't seem right because her feedings were solely breast milk. And she was feeding poorly. Some days, she didn't poop at all. Then she started vomiting every time she was fed. I thought she was constipated, so my husband, Ike, drove us to see our pediatrician, who told us to take her to the hospital."

Ike drove Blessing and Zara to the Howard University Hospital and dropped them off at the Emergency Room. It was late in the afternoon on Tuesday, March 2, 2021. The ER team examined Zara and agreed with Blessing. They thought Zara was constipated and gave her something for her stool. Overall, though, they thought she looked pretty good. Before leaving the ER, Blessing remembered to point out Zara's tense anterior fontanelle. That got the attention of the medical team, and they ordered an immediate CT scan of the head.

By now, it was early in the evening, and things began to happen quickly. Thinking back, Blessing feels her memory was blurred at the time. The ER team brought her into a room and asked her to have a seat. They told her the CT had been completed. Everyone looked somber, and Blessing knew there was something serious going on.

"Your baby has a mass," the doctor told her. "She has a large tumor in her brain. We are going to transfer her to Johns Hopkins right away."

"The news hit me like a bomb," Blessing recalled. "It was like a bad dream, a nightmare. I was all alone. It was the height of COVID-19. They asked me if there was anyone I wanted to call, and I called my husband, Ike, and gave him the news. He was a few miles away at home with my son Chuka. He jumped in the car with Chuka and came to the hospital immediately."

Meanwhile, the ER team at Howard had packed up Zara in an ambulance with the emergency medical technicians and immediately shipped her off to Johns Hopkins. By the time Ike and Chuka reached the hospital, Zara was already gone. Because of COVID-19 restrictions, Blessing wasn't allowed to ride with her in the ambulance. So, Ike drove Blessing to Johns Hopkins, dropped her off, and then returned home with Chuka. Full

COVID-19 visitor restrictions were in effect, and only one parent was allowed to be present in the Hopkins Children's Hospital. In the Adult Tower of Johns Hopkins Hospital, things were even worse—no visitors were allowed at all. The pandemic had created an emotional nightmare for patients and their families.

Blessing met up with the Hopkins pediatric neurosurgery team in the ER, where Zara was already being evaluated. She had become progressively more lethargic and was taken immediately to the OR, where my partner, Dr. Shenandoah Robinson, made a small opening in her skull on the right side and inserted a catheter into her lateral ventricle. The intracranial pressure was very high and came down when they drained some cerebrospinal fluid. Zara's mental status improved, and she was admitted to the pediatric intensive care unit (PICU).

I met Zara and her mother in the PICU early the next morning. Zara had been extubated the previous evening after the ventricular drain had been placed. She was more alert in the morning and more comfortable. Her anterior fontanelle was softer. But she still appeared stunned and was not normal.

Blessing was clearly on edge. She was able to pull herself together and ask appropriate questions.

"What happens next? My tiny baby has a large brain tumor. Where is it located? What are you going to do? What is the chance of survival?"

I wondered, as I often do in circumstances like this, how I would respond if I were in her shoes and it was one of my children in the PICU bed. Blessing was a courageous young woman, fiercely dedicated to helping bring her beloved infant daughter through this terrible ordeal. There's no way I would have been as poised and strong.

I showed Blessing the CT. "It's a big tumor in the cerebellum at the base of the brain," I said, pointing to the large mass on the right side of Zara's posterior fossa, crossing over to the left side, compressing the fourth ventricle, causing hydrocephalus. I noted to myself that the tumor was even larger than the normal cerebellum. "I think it's an aggressive tumor, most likely a form of brain cancer. Zara will need surgery so that we can diagnose the tumor and remove as much as is safely possible. But first, we need to do more studies, including an MRI of the brain and entire spine without and with contrast to get a more accurate picture and see if there's been any spread. There's no question this is a serious problem. But Zara has perked up nicely after the ventricular drain, and that's a good sign. We are going to hit the tumor with everything we have."

In matters like this, there's always a delicate balance between honesty and hope. Hearing that your infant child has been diagnosed with a malignant brain tumor is a gut-wrenching experience for anyone. Statistics can be stark, scary, and overwhelming. But sugarcoating the situation is never helpful. The goal is not to offer false hope—that can backfire and lead to erosion of trust between the doctor, patient, and family. Compassionate honesty is the goal. But taking away hope is a cardinal sin.

The MRI was impressive. The tumor was enormous and caused extensive mass effect on the normal brain structures, forcing the inferiorly located normal cerebellar tonsils down through the foramen magnum, the large opening in the skull base, causing crowding and compression of the brainstem. It was largely solid, with internal regions of hemorrhage and small cysts. The tumor encased the right vertebral artery, a major vessel supplying blood to the brain, and there were multiple other blood vessels within the substance of the tumor. It extended over the midline to compress the left vertebral artery. It enhanced after the administration of intravenous gadolinium contrast, and it restricted diffusion. The clinical presentation and radiographic findings suggested that this was a highly malignant tumor. The ventricular drain that had been inserted when Zara was admitted was in a good position, and the hydrocephalus looked a little improved.

An MRI of the spine showed evidence of leptomeningeal spread. The leptomeninges are the inner two linings of the brain, the arachnoid and pia mater. They lie just underneath the firm outer lining of the brain, the dura mater (Latin for "tough mother"). This signifies that Zara's posterior fossa brain tumor in her cerebellum had already metastasized to the spinal cord and spinal nerve roots. Additionally, there was an area of presyrinx in the cervical spinal cord, a collection of cerebrospinal fluid that was cavitating the spinal cord due to the blockage caused by the fact that the brain tumor had herniated through the foramen magnum and clogged the normal cerebrospinal fluid pathways.

For a neurosurgeon, the MRI findings represented a five-alarm fire. A picture like this is one of the worst-case scenarios one can imagine: a large hypervascular brain tumor in a young infant that has already spread outside the brain along the nervous system down to the spinal cord. I reviewed the films with our colleagues in neuroradiology and spent a considerable amount of time with my team developing a surgical plan.

We operated on Zara early in the morning on Thursday, March 4, 2021. She was seven months old. Blessing accompanied Zara to the OR and stayed by her side and cried as the anesthesia team put her to sleep. She later told me she remembers being overcome by fear. She felt that Zara was too tiny for the big procedure she was about to undergo. She didn't know if her daughter was going to live. She was wobbly on her feet as the circulating nurse escorted her to the waiting room.

As we set up the equipment in the OR, we shared Blessing's concerns. Our apprehension was the possibility of massive intraoperative bleeding in such a young infant. It was a complex operation, and I was working with two very experienced neurosurgeons, my fellow Jignesh Tailor and another of my partners, Eric Jackson. Our anxiety level was high. In some cases, when we operate on young children with very vascular malignant brain tumors, we do a small procedure to take a biopsy and then use neoadjuvant (up front) chemotherapy to alter the tumor by making it firmer and more fibrous, thereby cutting down its blood supply. This can sometimes work very nicely, allowing us to go back later and resect the tumor with less concern about intraoperative bleeding. But we couldn't do that in Zara's case because the tumor was so large that it was causing significant compression on her brainstem. We needed to debulk the tumor to get rid of that pressure.

We positioned Zara prone with her head supported by a padded horseshoe support and her neck flexed in a military tuck position to provide us maximal access to the tumor at the base of her brain. Before starting the case, we had blood in the room ready to be transfused. We gave Zara intravenous dexamethasone, a steroid, and cefazolin, an antibiotic. We also administered intravenous tranexamic acid (TXA), an antifibrinolytic agent that slows the breakdown of blood products and helps to mitigate bleeding.

We made a midline incision in the back of Zara's head, taking care to deepen the exposure by going through the avascular fibrous midline band. When we reached the skull, there was significant bleeding coming through the bone from large emissary veins because of the significantly elevated intracranial pressure from the tumor. We controlled this bleeding using a synthetic paste of bone wax, an ingenious material developed by Victor Horsley in the late nineteenth century, to plug the vascular holes in the bone. Horsley was a brilliant though eccentric pioneer neurosurgeon working at the National Hospital for Paralysis and Epilepsy at Queen Square in London, England. His original bone wax was a mixture of beeswax, salicylic acid, and almond oil. We now use a synthetic analog of Horsley's bone wax, which is very effective in controlling bleeding.

It's hard to imagine how the early neurosurgical pioneers could even think of doing brain surgery without bone wax, because bone bleeding can be significant and is difficult to control. Among multiple other contributions to the field of neurosurgery, Horsley was the first to remove a spinal cord tumor. He was also the first to perform a craniotomy for epilepsy. In fact, when his own teenage son Siward developed seizures and surgery was recommended, Horsley considered himself the most proficient to perform it, and carried out the surgery himself, though it did not cure the seizures. Later in life, Horsley volunteered as a field surgeon for the British Army in World War I and died unexpectedly of heat stroke in Iraq at the age of fifty-nine.

Next, we elevated a bilateral posterior fossa craniotomy, removing part of the base of the skull to expose the fibrous dura mater covering both cerebellar hemispheres. The dura was quite full because of the large size of the underlying tumor, so we drained some cerebrospinal fluid from the indwelling ventricular catheter and administered intravenous mannitol, a diuretic, to help bring down the elevated intracranial pressure. We also asked anesthesia to hyperventilate Zara in a further attempt to bring down the pressure in her head by blowing off carbon dioxide, thereby narrowing the arterial blood supply to the brain to reduce blood flow and help bring down the intracranial pressure. The measures worked, but only to a limited extent because the tumor was so large.

We identified the architecture and geometry of the tumor using transdural ultrasonography (sonar) and frameless stereotactic computer guidance. We opened the dura in a cruciate fashion, using small silver clips to control bleeding from a large occipital sinus, which is often present in young kids and can cause a lot of blood loss unless it is dealt with effectively. Although bleeding from this sinus is venous in nature and not arterial, it can be massive. In spite of all these carefully thought-out prophylactic measures, the brain began to herniate out of the head because of pressure from the underlying tumor.

To say that the surgery was nerve-wracking is an understatement. We had to work quickly and brought in the operating microscope. The tumor was red, rubbery, and extremely vascular. We debulked the tumor using a bipolar coagulator and suction catheter, along with topical hemostatic agents and pressure to control the profuse bleeding, while the anesthesia team transfused Zara and kept her hemodynamically stable, maintaining a good pulse and blood pressure. After working for several hours, we finally got the tumor out and closed, leaving a tiny portion that was stuck to Zara's brainstem, which we felt was unsafe to meddle with. The frozen section was a malignant embryonal tumor. That was no surprise to us. That's a highly aggressive brain cancer. We sent the rest of the resected tumor off for further analysis, including special histological stains and molecular and genetic profiling.

Zara's blood loss during the surgery was 250 milliliters—almost half of her circulating blood volume. Fortunately, the anesthesia team was able to keep her hemodynamically stable by administering intravenous fluids and transfusing packed red blood cells and fresh frozen plasma. Because of the complexity of the case, we left Zara intubated and sent her for a follow-up MRI, which showed postoperative changes but no evidence of residual bleeding. We brought her to the PICU.

Meanwhile, Blessing had spent the day in the waiting room, crying and praying. "It was the longest day of my life," she recalled.

Because we performed Zara's surgery in the middle of the COVID-19 pandemic, only one parent was allowed in the hospital. So, Blessing sat alone in the waiting room while Ike and Chuka stayed in their car in the hospital garage. It was an emotional nightmare for the Ilobi family and for other families whose children were hospitalized at the time. It wasn't enough that her daughter had to undergo surgery to remove a giant brain tumor, but Blessing had to endure the entire experience—preoperative, intraoperative, and postoperative—alone, separated from her husband and older son.

After surgery, I met up with Blessing at Zara's bedside in the PICU and told her what we had found. It had been a long day. The conversation was solemn. Zara had an aggressive brain cancer that had already spread throughout her nervous system. After a long seven-hour operation, she was still intubated and not awake. Blessing had tears in her eyes as she stood beside her motionless daughter in the PICU surrounded by a team of doctors, nurses, and a series of sterile bags on IV poles delivering fluids and medication into Zara's veins.

But there was reason to hope. Zara had made it through the surgery. Her vital signs were stable. The post-op MRI showed that the pressure on her brain and brainstem had been relieved. We needed to focus on helping her recover from the big procedure.

We removed Zara's endotracheal tube later in the day after the MRI was completed. She woke up and was able to interact with her mother, who would stay at her bedside every day around the clock. Zara talked and was able to move her arms and legs. But the next day, her breathing was labored. Her voice was softer, and she had trouble swallowing her oral secretions. We consulted the ENT team, who performed flexible laryngoscopy at the bedside and found partial paralysis of the right vocal cord. This was caused either by injury during surgery to the vagus, one of the lower cranial nerves as it exited the brainstem, or by trauma from the intubation. Zara's airway function stabilized, and the vagal nerve paralysis resolved completely after several months, suggesting it was likely caused by the irritation from the intubation for her anesthesia.

But Zara continued to have a stormy course after surgery. We tried to wean her external ventricular drain by slowly raising the pop-off for drainage. Our hope was that now that the tumor had been decompressed and her pathways had been opened, she would be able to absorb the normal daily half quart of cerebrospinal fluid she made. But as we raised the drainage pop-off, Zara became lethargic, and a repeat MRI showed that she had developed hydrocephalus, presumably related to scarring of the cerebrospinal fluid channels after surgery, even though the tumor had been removed.

So, a week after the tumor resection surgery, we took out the external ventricular drain and placed an internal ventriculoperitoneal shunt, which led to symptomatic improvement. Zara was able to swallow but required a nasogastric tube for feedings in order to get adequate nutrition. This was converted to a gastrostomy tube placed percutaneously, through the skin into the stomach, to continue feedings. The gastrostomy tube was ultimately removed after several months when Zara was able to tolerate full oral feedings.

Pathology returned atypical teratoid/rhabdoid tumor (AT/RT) with loss of *SMARCB1/INI-1* expression. Methylation profiling done by the National Institutes of Health confirmed the diagnosis and placed it in the TYR subclass. The description of this and other brain tumors in the most recent classification scheme used by the World Health Organization is daunting and sounds like an alphabet soup. But there is a method to the madness. The reason for the new classification is based on advances in molecular biology and genetics that enable scientists to look for specific mutations that can potentially be targeted with drugs that are more potent and less toxic than conventional chemotherapy.

The AT/RT is one of the most lethal cancerous tumors of the nervous system. It is extremely rare, with only about seventy new cases each year in the United States. It was first identified in 1987 as a cerebellar mass in a three-month-old infant boy who died two weeks after admission to the hospital. AT/RT usually occurs in infants and arises from embryonal cells left over from fetal development in the womb. It is a highly aggressive, fast-growing cancer with a dismal prognosis. The overall survival is less than a year from the time of diagnosis, though recent clinical trials have shown improved survival with novel combination therapy that includes radiation and multi-agent chemotherapy.

AT/RTs are caused by an inactivating mutation on the tumor suppressor gene, *SMARCB1/INI-1,* which is located on the long arm of chromosome 22. Recently, AT/RTs have been further classified into three subtypes. The subclass of Zara's tumor is TYR, meaning that it overexpresses tyrosinase, a copper-containing enzyme responsible for the first step in the synthesis of the pigment melanin. The significance of the TYR subclass of AT/RT is still being investigated. The TYR subclass of AT/RT is more likely to occur in young children under the age of one year and is more likely to occur in the posterior fossa of the skull, as was the case with Zara's tumor. There is hope that in the future, specific agents can be developed to target the tyrosinase enzyme and improve the efficacy of treatments.

Dr. Eric Raabe and the oncology team took over Zara's care. We discussed her case in our multidisciplinary tumor board and determined that she would be best treated with a combination of multi-agent chemotherapy and radiation. She underwent placement of a long-term Hickman catheter, a soft tube placed through the chest into the subclavian vein that comes out of the body for external access in order to deliver the chemotherapy in a sterile fashion.

Two weeks after her surgery, Zara began chemotherapy according to the ACNS0333 protocol of the Children's Oncology Group. This started with induction therapy using multiple high-powered intravenous agents, consisting of vincristine, methotrexate, etoposide, cyclophosphamide, and cisplatin. The idea behind this is to use heavy-duty chemotherapy drugs, each with a different mechanism of action, to kill the cancer cells. But these drugs are myeloablative (suppress the bone marrow activity) and also wipe out the patient's normal blood cells. So, the oncologists harvest stem cells from the patient and grow them in culture so that they can be replaced to reconstitute the normal blood cells.

The treatment regimen is highly toxic to both the tumor and the patient. Before her stem cell rescue, Zara's chemotherapy caused her to be pancytopenic, meaning that the drugs wiped out her red blood cells, white blood cells, and platelets. She developed a high fever, tachycardia (rapid heart rate), tachypnea (rapid respiratory rate) with respiratory distress, stridor (high-pitched noisy breathing), and copious tracheal secretions. This was caused by multi-drug-resistant bacteremia (blood infection) with *Pseudomonas aeruginosa*, a gram-negative rod that has a predilection for causing infection in immunocompromised hosts. Zara was immunocompromised from chemotherapy-induced neutropenia (reduced white blood cell count). The blood infection was accompanied by multifocal pneumonia with lung abscess formation.

This was a major problem requiring Zara to be brought back to the PICU, where she was intubated, placed on a mechanical ventilator, and treated with intravenous antibiotics. Her tube feedings had to be discontinued for a time, and she had to receive feedings intravenously by TPN—total parenteral nutrition. It was a horrible situation. Zara had lost weight and was unresponsive while she was sedated so that she could be maintained on the mechanical ventilator, because her own lung function was not adequate. She appeared deathly ill.

In the midst of Zara's chemotherapy, Blessing's mother died, also in Nigeria. Once again, she had to miss the funeral because Zara was so ill. The times were not easy for the Ilobi family.

Blessing was despondent. She had begun this journey with Zara with hope in her heart but became distressed when she saw Zara back in the PICU in such dire straits. She felt as if her prayers had gone unanswered. It was hard for her to watch what Zara was going through. She asked the medical team if we could let her daughter die peacefully.

I must admit I was having the same thoughts as Blessing. In the field of medicine, we undergo a lot of advanced training to enable us to care for sick patients. And we are intensely focused on preserving life. But there comes a time when the treatment can turn out to be worse than the disease. I wondered if we had reached that point with Zara. This was a lethal disseminated cancer. She had a galloping bacterial infection in the blood and lungs. She was an infant girl, unresponsive on a respirator, whose bone marrow had been destroyed by the medications being used to save her. Our neurosurgical team and I turned to Eric Raabe and asked if it was time to call off therapy and let nature take its course.

"No, let's just stay the course," Raabe said calmly. "This whole infection thing is because her blood counts were knocked out by the chemotherapy. Let's continue to support her a little longer. Her counts will come back. She'll fight the infection. Let's give her a chance to grow up."

I told him I thought he was delusional and that pediatric neuro-oncologists must always see the world through rose-colored lenses. They are eternal optimists. But Raabe was right. We followed his suggestion and continued supportive treatment for Zara. And her blood counts came back. She was able to fight the infection, get off the ventilator, and get out of the PICU. That was a turning point in Zara's treatment. It was a sight to behold. Kids are remarkably resilient. Blessing's hope returned, and so did mine. I was moved by the strength of Blessing's ironclad commitment to help her daughter fight this horrible disease. She was a truly courageous woman. I thought of the words of Theodore Roosevelt, who said, "Courage is not having the strength to go on, it is going on when you don't have the strength." Blessing's courage surely helped me to muster the strength to continue the fight.

Zara got out of the PICU and back on track. Her treatment continued with three cycles of consolidation chemotherapy using the intravenous agents thiotepa and carboplatin, along with peripheral blood stem cell rescue. This was not an easy regimen to tolerate, and Zara had several bouts of sepsis related to chemotherapy-induced neutropenia. At one point, her Hickman central venous catheter became infected and had to be removed and subsequently replaced after her blood counts came back up and her infection came under control.

But there was still that light at the end of the tunnel. Zara became more alert and playful, sitting upright, smiling, laughing, and clapping her hands, with significant improvement in her neurological exam. And her residual brain tumor shrank dramatically in size.

The next step for Zara was radiation therapy, which began when she was only fifteen months old. This was administered under the direction of Sahaja Acharya, our chief of Pediatric Radiation Oncology at Johns Hopkins. She is extremely smart, and her patients all adore her. But the treatment was arduous for little Zara.

Because the tumor had already spread throughout the nervous system to her spinal cord at the time of presentation, Zara would need craniospinal radiation. Radiation is toxic to the tumor but can also be toxic to the nervous system, particularly when the patient is a young child. Radiation therapy can cause cognitive dysfunction, psychosocial issues, endocrine problems, vascular disorders, alopecia, hearing loss, and even the formation of secondary tumors. To mitigate these complications, we chose to treat Zara with a gentler technique of proton beam radiotherapy. Protons are charged particles generated by a cyclotron that deliver only a small amount of energy along their path, releasing a large amount of energy at the end, the so-called Bragg peak, when they reach their target.

The proton beam therapy was administered five days a week for six weeks. Zara received thirty-six gray of radiation to the brain and spinal cord, with a boost to fifty-four gray to the tumor bed at the base of the brain. That's a healthy dose for anyone, particularly a tiny fifteen-month-old child. One gray is equal to the absorption of one joule of ionizing radiation energy per kilogram of body matter. This standard unit of radiation dosage was named for Louis Harold Gray, an English physicist who defined it, working at the Mount Vernon Hospital in northern London, England.

The Johns Hopkins Children's Hospital is in Baltimore, but the Proton Center is at the Johns Hopkins Sibley Memorial Hospital in Washington, DC. So, for every day of the one-hour proton beam treatments, Blessing had to drive her daughter an hour each way. And for each treatment, Zara had to be sedated with propofol. It was a complex logistical ordeal. However, with Zara improving clinically, hope had returned to Blessing's heart, and she made the trips without any complaints despite the heavy urban traffic on the roads.

The final stage of treatment for Zara was metronomic chemotherapy, in which equally spaced (metronomic) low doses of multiple oral agents are administered chronically to provide strong antineoplastic activity with minimal toxicity. At the same time, the oncologists wanted Zara to receive intrathecal chemotherapy with the agent topotecan, directly into the cerebral ventricles. Topotecan works by inhibiting the action of the enzyme topoisomerase, thereby killing tumor cells by damaging their DNA and really giving the tumor a run for its money.

Therefore, on February 18, 2022, when Zara was nineteen months old, we went back to the OR and inserted a right frontal Ommaya reservoir. The device was developed in 1963 by Ayub Khan Ommaya, a Pakistani American neurosurgeon who was also a Rhodes scholar and a trained opera singer. He would often regale his patients with song after completing a case, earning himself the nickname of the "singing neurosurgeon."

The Ommaya reservoir is a practical implant that contains a subcutaneous reservoir connected to a catheter whose tip goes into the lateral ventricle of the brain. After a sterile prep, a needle can be inserted into the reservoir through the scalp at the bedside to sample cerebrospinal fluid and inject medication, in this case, topotecan, into the ventricle. We had already placed a separate ventriculoperitoneal shunt in Zara a year earlier to control her hydrocephalus. That shunt had a special valve that enabled us to turn off the shunt for an hour using a magnet placed over Zara's scalp while the drug was infused. The shunt could then be turned on magnetically after the topotecan had been given a chance to work. These Ommaya reservoir treatments were all done monthly while Zara was an outpatient.

At one point, the day following one of the intrathecal injections, Blessing brought Zara to the emergency room. She was lethargic, and there was a collection of fluid under her scalp adjacent to the shunt reservoir. It wasn't clear what was going on until we placed a magnet over the shunt valve and found that it was still turned off. Apparently, when the doctor turned the shunt back on with the magnet, the shunt valve was stuck and didn't really turn back on. Zara needed the shunt to control her hydrocephalus. When the shunt was off for a day, the cerebrospinal fluid began to cause her ventricles to enlarge, and the fluid began to leak around the ventricular catheter and accumulate in her scalp. It was lucky that Heather Kerber, our physician assistant, recognized this because it could have turned into a big problem. It's often the simple things that can cause big problems. In this case, the solution was also simple: we turned the shunt valve back on with the magnet, and everything got better.

Zara was an incredible fighter throughout the long ordeal of adjuvant chemotherapy and radiation. She completed her metronomic oral chemotherapy on December 18, 2023. Her white blood cell and platelet counts were normal. Her hemoglobin was slightly low but would come back up to normal on its own. Two months later, on February 12, 2024, Zara received her last dose of intraventricular topotecan through her Ommaya reservoir, which she tolerated well. Her MRI showed no evidence of progression of her brain or spinal cord tumors. She was in remission. It had been a long haul for a little three-year-old girl: two brain surgeries followed by two years of heavy-duty radiation therapy to the brain and spinal cord and intravenous and intraventricular chemotherapy.

And after the long, drawn-out battle with disseminated brain cancer, Zara was the picture of health. If you saw her, you wouldn't believe what she had been through. She was eating well and had gained back all the weight she had lost. She was walking and talking and smiling when she rang the bell on the oncology floor, signifying completion of her therapeutic regimen. She was wearing a beautiful shirt with a floral design and matching pants, black sneakers, an oversized wristwatch, a bright red headband, and a pair of slightly tinted designer eyeglasses with a pink heart-shaped frame. Around her neck hung a gold band that held a gold medallion that matched the gold bell she proudly rang. She had a smile from ear to ear matched only by the smile of her mother, Blessing, who stood by her on that day, as she had every single day for the past two grueling years.

Today, Zara is a ray of sunshine. She remains in remission on no medication. She is in kindergarten, where she is reading and spelling. She is extroverted and loves to play with her friends. She loves to sing and dance, even when there's no music playing. She loves to run around at the park and hates to go back indoors. She enjoys spending time with her brother Chuka but fights with him frequently because she doesn't like to share her toys. Blessing still spends every day with her daughter, but the circumstances are vastly different from the two years of hell she had been through.

It's hard to find the words to convey the amount of emotion that was in the room on February 12, when Zara rang that bell. There is no love stronger than that of a mother for her young child, particularly after a years-long arduous battle with a lethal brain tumor. There were probably more than one hundred health-care providers who helped Zara on her journey. And no one is more dedicated than her mother, Blessing, with whom we rejoice at the good news of today and face a future of uncertainty with hope in our hearts.

CHAPTER 12

Resilience

"Hardships often prepare ordinary people for an extraordinary destiny."

C. S. Lewis

Sunday, December 10, 2006, was a cold and cloudy day in Slavic Village, one of the oldest neighborhoods in Cleveland, Ohio. But that didn't faze young Treasure Byrge in the slightest. She was fully engaged in a playdate with her younger sister, Trinity, and their Shetland Sheepdog, Wishbone. Their mother, Carol, brought in some rocks from the backyard for them to paint. Treasure was the picture of health. She had enjoyed celebrating her tenth birthday the week before with her family and classmates from school.

But things would take a drastic change the following day. It began routinely when Carol dropped Treasure off at Saint Stanislaus School, where she was in the fourth grade. Treasure was perfectly well, her usual chipper, jovial self. She had never really been sick before. But as the morning went on, things took a turn for the worse. Treasure began feeling dizzy. At about 10 a.m., when she was in the locker room suiting up for gym class, she developed the sudden onset of a severe progressive thunderbolt headache. As she was walking into the gym, a teacher saw she was pale and wobbly and took her into the bathroom, where she had repeated bouts of dry heaves.

The school had called Carol earlier in the morning and asked her to come pick up her daughter and bring her home because she appeared ill. Shortly after that, Treasure collapsed on the gym floor and became unresponsive. Carol hurried to the school and was surprised to see an ambulance and a fire truck in front of the building. She became terrified when she saw two emergency medical technicians (EMTs) wheeling Treasure out on a gurney, pale and unconscious.

They rushed her to nearby MetroHealth Medical Center. Carol left her car at the school and rode with Treasure and the two EMTs in the back of the ambulance. She remembers the two of them arguing back and forth, one saying that Treasure was in a coma, the other saying she wasn't. Then she heard one whisper to the other that maybe they shouldn't be having this conversation in front of the mother. But by then, Carol had already concluded that Treasure had to be in a coma because she wouldn't open her eyes or move in response to voices or painful stimuli.

In the Metro emergency room, the medical team agreed with Carol. Treasure was intubated and taken for a stat CT scan, which showed a massive hemorrhage in the center of her brain, along with hydrocephalus and blood in the enlarged cerebral ventricles. The neurosurgeons there performed an urgent lifesaving procedure right in the emergency room, placing a ventricular drain to control her markedly elevated intracranial pressure. To do this, they made a small twist drill hole on the left side of her skull and passed a thin catheter into the dilated ventricular system of her brain. Her intracranial pressure was sky high but came down slightly after they drained bloody cerebrospinal fluid. Unfortunately, she didn't awaken or improve neurologically.

The neurosurgery attending from Metro called me, told me the story, and immediately sent her by Life Flight helicopter to us at Rainbow Babies and Children's Hospital. Carol flew with her daughter and the medical team in the helicopter. She was scared. Her little girl had been completely normal a few hours earlier when she dropped her off at school. "Now I was terrified that my Treasure was going to die," Carol said. She held Treasure's hand during the flight and spoke to her in a comforting voice even though Treasure was unconscious.

I met them in the emergency room at Rainbow. It was clear that Treasure was seriously ill. Her deterioration had been extremely rapid and was likely the result of the sudden hemorrhage deep in the ventricles of the brain. But what caused the hemorrhage? Healthy kids don't bleed spontaneously. Was there an underlying lesion that bled? There was nothing in her history to suggest she ever had a problem before this. We needed to get more imaging studies quickly before planning any further surgical intervention.

In the differential diagnosis of what was going on, the two leading possibilities were a bleed from a ruptured arteriovenous malformation (AVM), an abnormal tangle of blood vessels in the brain that she might have been born with, or a bleed into a brain tumor. Both conditions are serious, but their management is very different. We would need an MRI and a cerebral angiogram (blood vessel X-ray of the brain) to better delineate the problem.

So that's exactly what we did. The MRI showed a large hemorrhagic mass in the hydrocephalic right lateral ventricle that had crossed the midline into the left lateral ventricle. Most of the blood was in an organized blob deep in the center of the brain, but there was also free blood mixing with the cerebrospinal fluid in the ventricles. The MRI also gave a nice demonstration of the geometry of the lesion and its relationship to vital structures adjacent to it. The cerebral angiogram showed no obvious abnormal arteries or veins to suggest an AVM. So, our working diagnosis was that Treasure's sudden neurologic deterioration was caused by a hemorrhage into a deep-seated brain tumor in the middle of her head.

That's a rare occurrence and usually happens when the tumor is malignant (cancerous). So, we brought Treasure to the PICU, stabilized her with medication, and I sat down with Carol to make a plan. Despite the ventricular drainage, the large mass in the center of her head was still causing dangerous pressure on the brain. She would need to undergo further surgery to remove the mass.

Carol was a mess. Everything had happened so suddenly. She had no time to process what was going on. She was a single parent and had never faced a health-care crisis like this. Here I was, a complete stranger, telling her that her daughter needed emergency brain surgery. She didn't know whether she could trust me. Was she making the right decision? I had just come out of the OR after a long case and was wearing wrinkled surgical scrubs and white clogs with no socks. Years later, she would tell me that she had no idea who I was and thought I looked like some fashion-insensitive yahoo. Sadly for me, that was not the first time I'd heard a sentiment like that, in both my professional and personal life.

Carol asked if she could get another opinion. I told her I would be happy to speak with anyone, but the clock was ticking, and there wasn't time for a formal outside consultation. I went over the OR plan step by step and tried to calm her. She was paralyzed with fear and couldn't make a decision. Finally, in a soft but firm, composed, serious voice, I said, "If we don't do the surgery, I don't think Treasure will survive."

Carol consented immediately. Those were not easy words for a mother to hear. I thought about my own two young boys, who were similar in age to Treasure. That's one of the challenges for pediatric neurosurgeons with young children. It brings a uniquely personal perspective to the critical illnesses we deal with. While it may help us empathize with the families of our patients, it's hard for me to think about how I would handle things if my own child were the patient.

By now, it was Monday evening. It had been a long day. We continued to bring down Treasure's intracranial pressure by removing CSF from her ventricular drain and using medication. Our plan was to wait another day before the craniotomy to allow her angry, swollen brain to cool down with the external ventricular drainage.

The next morning, Carol came to visit me in my office. She was more composed and spoke to me in the waiting room in earshot of my assistant, Helen, and several families who were sitting there waiting to see me.

"Dr. Cohen, tomorrow you are operating on my daughter. I need you to be at your best. Please promise me you won't have sex tonight."

I was taken aback by her request and blushed. Surprisingly, though, that was not the first time I was asked that question before surgery. I tried to compose myself and said with a smile, "I thought that was only important for athletes." But I promised to comply.

We brought Treasure to the OR early in the morning on Tuesday, December 12, 2006. I did the surgery with my smart and good-natured senior resident, Andreas Tomac. We positioned Treasure supine on the OR table, shaved her head, and registered her to the computer guidance system to enable us to select the safest route to get to the deep-seated lesion in the brain.

In this case, we chose an interhemispheric transcallosal approach.[2] We made an incision across the scalp, opened the skull in the right frontal region with a quadrilateral bone flap right up to the midline, enabling us to go deep in the head in between the two hemispheres of the brain without having to traverse any essential tissue except a small amount of the corpus callosum, the white matter fiber bundle connecting the two cerebral hemispheres. The transcallosal approach is one of my favorite surgical procedures because the anatomy is so beautiful and because it allows us to get down to the deep, hidden structures using the operating microscope without traumatizing the brain.

Treasure's case was a little different than the standard elective transcallosal approach. She was rendered unconscious from the hemorrhage, and her brain was still under pressure, so we needed to move quickly but carefully as we peeled the two cerebral hemispheres apart. The anesthesia team hyperventilated Treasure, which blew off carbon dioxide, thereby narrowing the arteries to the brain, which helped to reduce the intracranial pressure. Once we opened the corpus callosum, we found the large hemorrhagic tumor in the lateral ventricles and began removing it using microsuction and bipolar cautery. Over several hours, we were able to get the tumor out and unblock the ventricles.

---

[2] Described in more detail in Chapter 3.

The pressure inside the brain subsided. We removed the ventricular drain that had been placed in the ER at MetroHealth Medical Center because of concern it might become infected, since it had been inserted in dire conditions. We replaced it with another ventricular drain, which we were subsequently able to wean and remove after a few days. We replaced the bone flap with titanium microplates and screws and closed Treasure up in routine fashion.

The intraoperative frozen section returned, suggesting a high-grade glioma (brain cancer) that had bled. That made sense because brain tumors that bleed spontaneously are more likely to be malignant, though that isn't always the case. We sent most of the brain tumor for special staining, and the final diagnosis would have to wait for a few days.

Meanwhile, Carol was pacing nervously in the waiting room, intermittently praying and watching TV to distract herself. Treasure had been in the OR for seven hours, but to Carol, it felt like forever. Carol's parents had made the four-hour drive from southern Ohio to be with her, and several friends came to the hospital as well. "We didn't know anything about brain surgery," she said, "but we all knew what was going on was a big deal."

Treasure was extubated at the end of the procedure and woke up a half hour later. Her first words to the bedside nurse were, "I want my mama."

I brought Carol to the PICU for an emotional reunion with her daughter. Treasure was awake, alert, talking coherently, and following commands. Treasure smiled. Carol cried. Treasure's eyes were swollen, and she had a big white turban on her head. She looked at herself in the mirror and was upset that the head-wrap made her look ugly. So, Carol went and found some magic markers and, with the flair of an artist, turned Treasure's head-wrap into a striking golden crown.

On the third post-op day, we removed the ventricular drain at the bedside and transferred Treasure out of the PICU to the floor. The swelling around her eyes had gone down. She was getting physical therapy and was able to walk around the ward and visit the game room. We started taking some of the IVs out of her arms.

Carol remained emotional, knowing that there was concern that her daughter might not have survived the ordeal. And not knowing what the final diagnosis would be. But Treasure was composed and appeared relaxed and low-key. "It's not the end of the world or anything, Mom. I'm gonna be fine," she said. We took the turban off, revealing her bald head and the scar we had made to do the surgery. Carol did a double-take and appeared dumbfounded by what she saw.

I tried to soften the blow and told Carol, "We placed the incision behind the hairline. So don't worry, when the hair grows back, you won't see it." For some reason, though, my words seemed to fall flat. Carol remained fixated and stunned. Then Treasure chimed in, "My hair's gonna grow back, Mom. It's no big deal. Don't sweat it." She was calm and collected as she sat up in bed next to a large stuffed animal puppy the medical staff had given her. Carol hugged her and smiled.

I was a little disconcerted. Didn't I essentially say the same thing? Weren't my words good enough? What would it take for me to finally earn Carol's trust? Actually, once Carol saw that her daughter had survived the surgery and was awake and talking, her nerves began to settle down. We were all pretty happy because Treasure was doing so well, and she continued to turn on the charm. Her resilience was infectious. Nothing seemed to faze her. Time and again, I've seen the same phenomenon with other patients—the strength of the child helping to comfort the parents as they navigated through troubled waters. The acclaimed Chilean American author Isabel Allende said it nicely, "We don't even know how strong we are until we are forced to bring that hidden strength forward."

The final pathologic diagnosis came back the same day Treasure was transferred out of the PICU, on post-op day three. That's an incredibly fast turnaround. The diagnosis was made by Dr. Mark Cohen (no relation), the director of neuropathology at the Case Western Reserve University School of Medicine. Mark is a brilliant neuropathologist, but one who marches to his own beat, playing guitar in a rock band in his spare time. The final diagnosis came as a big surprise to us. It was a glioneuronal neoplasm consistent with a subependymal giant cell astrocytoma (SEGA), with intratumoral hemorrhage.

That diagnosis was surprising for three reasons. First, a SEGA is not considered a malignant tumor, as we had initially suspected the tumor was going to be based on Treasure's clinical presentation, MR imaging, and the frozen section. SEGAs are considered benign, WHO grade 1 tumors. Second, although SEGAs are vascular tumors, they very rarely present with spontaneous intratumoral hemorrhage. Third, SEGAs are found almost exclusively in the setting of the unique neurocutaneous disorder, tuberous sclerosis. Neurocutaneous disorders affect the nervous system and skin, along with other organs. And there was no evidence whatsoever to suggest that Treasure had tuberous sclerosis.

SEGAs arise from the star-shaped supporting cells of the brain called astrocytes. They are usually found in the lateral ventricles near the foramen of Monro, the small opening between the lateral and third ventricles. When small, they are usually asymptomatic, but if they enlarge to obstruct the foramen of Monro, they can cause symptomatic hydrocephalus with headache, vomiting, lethargy, and even death from increased intracranial pressure.

SEGAs develop from benign, smaller subependymal nodules, histologically similar growths on the walls of the ventricles. They enlarge slowly. They are rare neoplasms, accounting for less than 1 percent of all intracranial tumors. They are more commonly seen in children, are often diagnosed in infancy, and usually occur in the first two decades of life. SEGAs get their name from the large swollen size of the giant astrocytes, called gemistocytes, with pink billowing cytoplasm.

It is extremely unusual for a patient with a SEGA to present with bleeding into the tumor. Only a handful of cases have been described worldwide. The tumors have a rich blood supply, but even so, spontaneous hemorrhage is an extremely rare occurrence. It's important for the treating team to remember that intratumoral hemorrhage in SEGAs is rare but can occur. Thus, SEGA should be considered in the differential diagnosis of intraventricular hemorrhage in a child, though it's lower down on the list. However, because the bleed is potentially lethal, rapid diagnosis and surgical evacuation can be lifesaving.

In most cases, SEGAs occur as a part of the genetic syndrome, tuberous sclerosis. Tuberous sclerosis is a rare disorder in which the child may develop noncancerous tumors of the nervous system and body, including the brain, eyes, skin, heart, kidneys, and lungs. It follows neurofibromatosis as the second most common neurocutaneous syndrome. Tuberous sclerosis is inherited in an autosomal dominant pattern. That is, an aberration of only a single non-sex chromosome is all that's necessary for a parent to pass on the syndrome to a child. The disorder can also occur sporadically.

Tuberous sclerosis, previously called Bourneville disease, is a fascinating disorder. It was discovered in the nineteenth century and named for Désiré-Magloire Bourneville, a neurologist working at the famous Hôpital Pitié-Sapêtrière in Paris, France. He cared for a fifteen-year-old girl with intellectual disability, seizures, and a vesico-papular eruption on her face who died in her bed on May 7, 1879, at 3 a.m. Bourneville performed an autopsy on his patient and found firm nodules in the cerebral cortex and tumors in the cerebral ventricles. He believed the potato-like sclerotic (hardened) areas on the surface of the brain were the cause of the patient's seizures and called them "sclérose tubéreuse des circonvolutions cérébrales," hence the name tuberous sclerosis, of the cerebral convolutions.

Previously, tuberous sclerosis was characterized by the triad of mental retardation, seizures, and bimalar facial angiofibromas (a pink butterfly rash on both cheeks). Over the years, we've learned a lot about the genetics of tuberous sclerosis. It has a prevalence of about 1/5,000 to 1/10,000 live births. There are about a million people with tuberous sclerosis worldwide. It's caused by a mutation in one of two tuberous sclerosis complex genes called *TSC1* (located on chromosome 9q) and *TSC2* (located on chromosome 16p). These are tumor suppressor genes that encode proteins called hamartin and tuberin, respectively, which act by regulating cellular growth. Mutation of the suppressor genes reverses their tumor suppressor effect and leads to tumorigenesis.

We now know that there are many more tuberous sclerosis features than the original triad described. And not all patients have all the findings. Some patients may show only some of the physical findings and may even be cognitively normal.

There are two main neurologic features of tuberous sclerosis. One is the SEGA, which can enlarge in the cerebral ventricles, causing hydrocephalus and increased intracranial pressure. The other is the cortical tuber, a firm, benign, potato-textured growth at the brain surface that can irritate the cerebral cortex and cause seizures. Other physical manifestations of tuberous sclerosis are cardiac rhabdomyomas (benign tumors of the heart), renal angiomyolipomas (benign tumors of the kidney), pulmonary lymphangioleiomyomas (overgrowth of tissue in the airways of the lungs), ash leaf spots (hypomelanotic macules of the skin), shagreen patches (firm raised eruptions of the skin mimicking the skin of a shark), and retinal hamartomas (benign tumor-like tissue in the back of the eye).

Five to 15 percent of children with tuberous sclerosis have SEGAs. So, when we diagnose a SEGA, we always undertake a search for tuberous sclerosis. And that's what we did with Treasure. Dr. Nancy Bass of pediatric neurology followed her with us and, along with our genetics team, outlined an extensive workup for tuberous sclerosis. The workup was negative. Treasure had no intellectual impairment. In fact, she was extraordinarily bright. She never had seizures. And there was no facial eruption on her cheeks. The only physical finding was a small, solitary ash leaf spot on one of her arms that was only noted during examination with a Wood's lamp, a special ultraviolet light developed by the American physicist, Robert Wood, used by dermatologists to help identify cutaneous lesions. That finding was not enough to make the diagnosis. Treasure was one of the rare children with a SEGA who didn't have tuberous sclerosis.

For someone like Treasure, who developed sudden neurological deterioration due to hemorrhage in the tumor, the treatment is urgent surgical decompression. For other symptomatic patients with SEGA, surgery is effective as well. Nowadays, there is also an opportunity for medical treatment, particularly if the tumor is in a tricky location that would make surgery riskier.

Recently, pharmacotherapy has been found to be effective in shrinking SEGAs, based on advances in molecular biology. SEGAs are driven by a unique biological pathway that controls growth and proliferation, called mammalian target of rapamycin, or mTOR. The tumor-suppressor genes, *TSC1* and *TSC2,* code for the proteins hamartin and tuberin, respectively. The way these proteins work is by inhibiting the mTOR pathway. Mutations in these genes prevent inhibition of the mTOR pathway and lead to growth of SEGAs.

The discovery of the drug rapamycin is an interesting story. Back in the 1960s, the government of Chile was planning to build an international airport on its property in the South Pacific, Easter Island. Easter Island is one of the most isolated islands in the world. A group of Canadian scientists organized a mission to go there to study the population and the impact that the airport would have once the islanders became exposed to the outside world.

As part of the mission, the scientists sampled the soil to elucidate the diversity of microorganisms on the island. By chance, the team identified a gram-positive aerobic bacterium in the soil, *Streptomyces hygroscopicus,* which acted as an antifungal agent. They gave it the name rapamycin, derived from the Polynesian name for the island, Rapa Nui. It was later found that rapamycin was also an immunosuppressant agent with powerful anticancer activity in humans. Rapamycin is even undergoing investigation as a possible anti-aging agent.

Administration of drugs that are mTOR inhibitors, such as sirolimus (rapamycin) and everolimus, can lead to shrinkage of SEGAs as well as other tuberous sclerosis tumors. These drugs are being used more frequently in selected SEGA cases in attempts to avoid the need for surgery. The medications, though promising, are expensive and not risk-free. Side effects include suppression of the immune system, oral inflammation, and high blood pressure. Furthermore, the tumors will start to grow again if the medication is ever stopped.

Meanwhile, Treasure continued to make a rapid recovery. She would sit up in her partially reclined bed, cool as a cucumber, with her hands behind her head, wearing her earrings, and wax philosophical with us. We learned a lot from her and admired her perpetual upbeat attitude. She told us how she was going to beat this tumor and get back to her life quickly. She received inpatient physical therapy and pushed herself hard to get back on her land legs. She got several visits from the pet therapy dogs. Santa came by to give her a hug.

Treasure was discharged from the hospital in good spirits just before Christmas. Channel 3, the local TV news station, did a heartwarming story about her for the holidays. The reporter, Lydia Esparra, movingly said, "The scar across her head is large, but her will to live is even larger. And in a world in which many are about to celebrate Christmas, Treasure is the jewel her family will be grateful to find in their stockings."

Carol beamed and replied tearfully, "I'm gonna put her under the tree when we get home. Because, yeah, she's the best Christmas present ever."

As soon as she left the hospital, Treasure got right back to work over the holiday break. She was incredibly organized and was able to make up all the lessons she'd missed in school while she was out. She was able to return to her fourth-grade class with all of her friends to start the new year in January, only a few weeks after her surgery. And she was also able to spend some time relaxing at home with family and friends before starting the new year. "There's a lot more joking and a lot more love in the family," Carol said. "Everybody knows what almost happened."

Treasure is a poster child for resilience. For her, the glass was always half full. And I think her mindset helped in her recovery. She came back to join us at Rainbow Babies and Children's Hospital for our annual Elvis Day celebration on January 8, to help mark the birthday of the King. That was a recurring ritual, when I would put on my rhinestone suit and bring my young patients up on the stage with me to sing karaoke songs for the patients and staff in the hospital (see Chapter 3).

At the time, Treasure was still freshly recuperating from her brain tumor resection. But that didn't stop her from assuming the role of lead dancer for our motley troupe. She was amazing. She was fearless. I was reminded of the German philosopher Friedrich Nietzsche's observation, "That which does not kill us makes us stronger." Treasure's courage and passion served as an inspiration for everyone in the room. She even brought her younger sister, Trinity, on stage with her and showed her how to dance like a rock star. Also on the stage with us was Treasure's neurologist, Dr. Nancy Bass, an extraordinary doctor and a gifted dancer with a great sense of humor. She shares a January 8 birthday with the King. What our group lacked in talent, we made up for with enthusiasm. It's a lighthearted, unconventional event to be sure, but a way to bring the kids, parents, and hospital staff together to promote healing.

Treasure went on to graduate with honors from Parma Senior High School in 2015. Four years later, she graduated from Walsh University in North Canton, Ohio, with honors in a double major of clinical psychology and occupational therapy. While in college, she did research with Professor Michael Decker in the Departments of Anatomy and Neuroscience at Case Western Reserve University, working in the Aerospace Physiology Research Laboratory. They collaborated with the United States Air Force to examine the effects of high altitude on oxygenation of the brain, analyzing changes in gray and white matter tracts on diffusion tensor imaging sequences of MRIs. It was surreal for me to imagine my former little ten-year-old fourth-grader bringing research patients to the same MRI machines that we used to diagnose her own brain tumor so many years earlier. She had really come full circle.

After college, Treasure was accepted into a highly competitive Public Health Associate Program Fellowship at the Centers for Disease Control and Prevention (CDC). She currently lives in Douglasville, Georgia, a suburb of Atlanta, with her life partner, Gabe. She serves as a public health adviser with the CDC in Atlanta and travels worldwide to help support the infrastructure of public health departments in other countries. In her spare time, she's earning a master's degree in public health at Georgia State University.

One pleasant perk about being an older pediatric neurosurgeon is that I am able to chart the course of my patients' lives over the years. Treasure told me recently that having had that near-tragic experience as a young child had a major impact on her and helped shape her way of thinking ever since. Even to this day, she faces life's challenges head-on with ambition, motivation, and strength. "Dealing with that brain tumor," she said, "taught me how to become more flexible and resilient in dealing with the problems I face now and in the future."

That reminds me of the words of the legendary New Zealand explorer Edmund Hillary, who, on May 29, 1953, with Tibetan Sherpa guide Tenzing Norgay, became the first to reach the summit of Mount Everest: "It's not the mountain we conquer, but ourselves."

CHAPTER 13

Hope

"Hope is the ability to see that there is light despite all the darkness."

Desmond Tutu
Former Archbishop of Cape Town, South Africa
Recipient of the Nobel Peace Prize, 1984

On the evening of Monday, February 7, 2022, I was working at my desk at Johns Hopkins Children's Hospital when I got a call from Aylin Tekes. Aylin was the chief of pediatric radiology, and it was unusual for her to call me in the evening unless there was a serious problem. I was already on the phone talking with a patient's family, and I text messaged her that I'd call her right back.

It had been a long day, and I was on edge, having finished a difficult case. I was multitasking at the time, looking at my computer while I was on the phone, and I realized that the world was on edge as well. President Emmanuel Macron of France was on a diplomatic mission in Moscow, meeting with President

Vladimir Putin of Russia in an attempt to ease the tensions of the European Union over Russia's military buildup around Ukraine. The meeting was strained, and a photo of the two men sitting twenty feet apart at opposite ends of a long oval table in a formal, ornate room forebode what was to come.

I had been paying little attention to current events, preoccupied with the complex surgical case I had performed earlier in the day, in which I removed a brain tumor from the left temporal lobe of a teenage boy named Daniel. The tumor had announced itself by causing a series of seizures over several weeks with focal shaking of his right arm. One spell was followed by generalized tonic-clonic (stiffening and shaking) activity of all limbs and transient loss of consciousness—a grand mal seizure. This prompted a neurologist to order a brain MRI, which lit up the tumor as a non-enhancing mass adjacent to his language center. Daniel was right-handed, and this was his dominant temporal lobe.

In an attempt to preserve his speech function during surgery, we decided to map the language center in his temporal lobe preoperatively with a functional MRI (fMRI). As expected, we found that it was directly adjacent to the tumor. The fMRI is a magnetic scan of the brain performed with the patient awake. During the scan, we ask the patient to look at pictures and name objects to enable us to locate electrical signals coming from the speech neurons. This electrical activity is monitored indirectly by measuring regional changes in blood flow as the patient talks to us. The technique is called BOLD—for blood-oxygenation-level-determination—and is helpful in selected OR cases when we work in areas of the eloquent brain, in this case, to protect speech.

In Daniel's case, we were concerned enough about the proximity of the tumor to his language fibers that we decided to do the operation as an awake craniotomy. An awake craniotomy enables us to interact with the patient during surgery as we electrically stimulate various areas of the brain to provide more precise localization of the speech area, in order to preserve it. It is a unique procedure that relies on the extraordinary cooperation of the patient with the OR team. It can seem unsettling to observe a patient lying on the OR table and talking to us with his skull open and his brain exposed. The reason we can do that is because the brain, the seat of all sensation, does not feel pain. There are pain fibers in the scalp and in the dural linings of the brain, which we can dampen with local anesthesia. Then we can work on the brain all we need to with the patient awake, without causing discomfort. Once we finish the localization and get our bearings, we can put the patient to sleep and take out the tumor.

We don't do many awake craniotomies in kids because the procedure requires absolute cooperation from the child, who must be awake and immobilized in a pin head holder. We chose to do the awake craniotomy for Daniel because he was bright, mature, and cooperative. It would offer extra protection to avoid injury to his language center. But Daniel became claustrophobic during the case and decided he wanted to get up and leave the OR, even though his skull was open and we hadn't resected the tumor yet. And his head was immobilized in pins! So, to avert disaster, we rapidly had to put him under general anesthesia for the rest of the procedure. Fortunately, our pre-op fMRI mapping was helpful enough, and we were able to complete the operation. The tumor proved to be a benign low-grade glioma, and he awoke from surgery able to speak, which was a great relief to us.

That's where my mind was when I got Aylin's call. I was anxiously awaiting Daniel's post-op MRI. The post-op MRI offers a stark appraisal of the success of surgery. In Daniel's case, I was concerned about the possibility of hemorrhage or swelling due to his sudden attempt to escape from the OR at an inopportune time. The MRI was done a bit later and thankfully looked okay. I was also the pediatric neurosurgeon on call that night and was awaiting the transfer of a child from another hospital with a head injury from a motor vehicle accident.

Aylin told me that Shivani Ahlawat, a senior radiologist at our medical center, had called about her nephew, who lived a few hundred miles away in New Jersey. He had just been diagnosed with a brain tumor. An MRI had been done that afternoon, and the diagnosis came as a complete surprise. The family was distraught. Shivani asked Aylin if she could speak to me. So, I called her.

Shivani was not a neuroradiologist, but she was an extremely bright and sophisticated radiologist. Her nephew Viaan, nicknamed Vinny, was seven years old and had developed some gait unsteadiness over several months. Shivani's husband, Ajay Hooda, was also medically sophisticated and served as the chief medical officer at another hospital in our city. Ajay was the brother of Vinny's father, Rahul Hooda.

Shivani had already obtained a digitized copy of the noncontrast MRI and was able to share it with me so we could review it together. It showed an irregularly round diffusion-restricting fourth ventricular brain tumor. We both immediately recognized the gravity of the situation. Shivani wanted Vinny to come to Johns Hopkins for treatment. She asked me to call her sister-in-law, Priyanka Hooda, Vinny's mother. So, I did.

It was 9 p.m. that night when I reached her on the phone. She had learned a few hours earlier that the doctors had found a mass on Vinny's MRI that was likely a brain tumor. She was terrified and tearful, sitting on the floor of her bedroom in shock. She had been packing boxes as the family was in the process of moving. Her parents were in the room, sitting on the bed, and her husband Rahul was also there, sitting on a chair nearby. Somehow, Priyanka managed to pull herself together as she told me the story.

Vinny had been a normal, healthy kid all his life. He was doing very well in first grade. About two months earlier, Priyanka saw that sometimes his right hand would be shaking. His handwriting had started to deteriorate. Months earlier, it had been perfect. Priyanka collected samples of his handwriting over the past several months, and it was clear that it had become significantly worse. She also observed that every day when Vinny came home from school, he had chocolate milk or a strawberry smoothie spilled all over his hoodie. She presumed this was related to his shaking right hand. Sometimes he walked as if he were drunk and would often bump into things. When she went to help him put on his pajamas, she saw his left hand flailing. She was concerned that there was something serious going on.

Priyanka became increasingly alarmed. She brought Vinny to see his pediatrician, who confirmed her suspicions and referred him to a child neurologist. Shivani, who had heard the story from Priyanka but hadn't seen Vinny, was concerned as well. She asked her husband, Ajay Hooda, to weigh in. Ajay, Rahul's brother, was Vinny's uncle. He was an internal medicine specialist who also served as the chief medical officer at his hospital. Ajay strongly recommended that Priyanka tell the neurologist that Vinny should have an MRI of his brain without and with contrast.

During his visit to the neurologist, Vinny looked pretty good. He was awake and appropriately interactive. He had no headache, and on ophthalmologic exam, there was no papilledema to suggest increased intracranial pressure. The neurologist thought that his symptoms were likely stress-related—the entire family was under a great deal of pressure at the time. Both parents were working full-time, and they were in the process of moving and closing on a new home. And Vinny and his older brother Veer, who was ten years old and in the fourth grade, would be switching schools mid-year. The neurologist didn't think an MRI would be necessary.

"Something is not right with my son," Priyanka said. "Can we just go ahead and get the MRI? My husband and I will sleep better." She wondered to herself if she was overreacting.

The neurologist ultimately acquiesced and agreed to order the MRI, but only without contrast. His level of suspicion for finding something was low, and he was aware of the potential risks associated with the administration of intravenous contrast. It was lucky that the neurologist chose not to ignore Priyanka's request. Her persistence would prove to be fortunate. If there's one thing I've learned over the years, it's to never ignore a mother's intuition. I believe the mother's insight is more than just intuition. It likely comes from close observation of her child and attentive, meticulous data-gathering. I've failed to take mother's words seriously more than once in my career, and I've regretted it every time.

Although a patient's mother doesn't always hold a medical degree, she knows more about her child than anyone else. She's with the child day in and day out and sees a longitudinal picture that is not available during a one-time exam at the doctor's office. It's one of the most important lessons I teach my trainees. Learn from my past mistakes. Listen to mom. She is almost always right.

The MRI was performed at a local health center in the afternoon on February 7. Vinny's parents both accompanied him to the scan. There was a lot going on that day. They had closed on their new home that morning, and there was a problem with the paperwork that had to be ironed out. Rahul had to leave before the scan was done to pick up his older son, Veer, from school. Priyanka stayed with Vinny, and the scan went smoothly. She brought him home an hour later.

The news was surprising and disturbing. Later that afternoon, Priyanka got a call from the neurologist, who told her that he was surprised to learn that the MRI showed a mass that appeared to be a brain tumor. He recommended an appointment with a pediatric neurosurgeon of his friend in New York City who could see Vinny in a few weeks. Priyanka was numb and didn't know what to do. She immediately called Shivani, who was able to get a copy of the scan and wanted Vinny to come to Johns Hopkins. Shivani got hold of Aylin Tekes, who put me in touch with Shivani and Priyanka that night.

That's what led to my late-night conversation with Priyanka as she sat on the floor of her bedroom surrounded by her family. It was a pleasant but somber conversation. Once again, I struggled to find the appropriate balance between honesty and hope.

I discussed the MRI findings and attempted to give something for Priyanka to hang on to. The mass on the scan did appear to be a tumor, and the restriction of diffusion suggested that it could be malignant. The positive news was that Vinny was in good shape neurologically, and there was no hydrocephalus. Controlled optimism is an essential part of patient care. Even in the worst-case scenario, in the modern era, there are several brain cancers that can be controlled and even cured.

"We need to do a few more studies, and then we need to get the tumor out," I said. "The sooner, the better. It's not doing anything good in there." It was only a ten-minute exchange, but

Priyanka and I had connected. I answered the family's questions, and we set up a visit for them to come see me.

I met Vinny and his parents in person a few days later. He was an adorable, engaging youngster who appeared perfectly normal at first glance. He was aware of his unsteadiness and walking difficulties. Otherwise, he felt fine. Specifically, he had no headache, nausea, or vomiting. When I examined him, the only remarkable findings were some dysmetria (uncoordinated movements) of his right arm and some truncal ataxia, a wide-based "drunken sailor" gait in which he tended to veer off to the right. This became particularly apparent when he was asked to tandem walk, heel-to-toe, in a straight line. Fundoscopic examination of the back of the eyes with an ophthalmoscope showed no papilledema, a reassuring sign along with his absence of headache, that there was likely no significant increased intracranial pressure.

The neurological exam pointed to an abnormality in the posterior fossa at the base of his brain involving the midline and right side of his cerebellum, the bottom part of the brain that modulates movement and balance. Neurologic diagnosis is a fascinating field, like detective work, in which the physician must act like an investigator to uncover the location and cause of the patient's problem. The wise clinician will begin to formulate a differential list of possible diagnoses based on the patient's chief complaint and description of the illness. Much can be learned from a thorough history followed by a detailed exam to confirm one's suspicions. Further diagnostic testing, including imaging studies, helps to confirm the diagnosis.

In this case, I had the advantage of already having seen the non-contrast MRI, which showed a tumor in the midline of the cerebellum going off to the right side. The MRI is a very powerful and noninvasive aid in neurologic diagnosis. As we look to the future, artificial intelligence (AI) is on the horizon and is moving fast with efforts to enhance diagnostic accuracy. But in the current era of advanced technology, there can be a tendency for the physician to underestimate the importance of bedside diagnosis. I believe we are already experiencing a lost art of localization as we come to rely more on ancillary tests, like CT and MRI. I've had patients referred to me with non-specific complaints—such as headaches and fatigue—that prompted workup with a total-body MRI. The problem with this kind of workup is that modern imaging studies are so advanced that the atypical shadows that they may identify are not always clinically significant.

With the availability of all of our sophisticated technology, there is still no substitute for a careful bedside history and physical exam. When searching for a diagnosis, it is tempting for the clinician to begin with a barrage of questions. A better plan is to talk less and listen more. The late Robert Buckman, a renowned oncologist from Princess Margaret Hospital in Toronto, recognized the importance of listening in patient care. He advised, "Before you talk, hear."

We physicians know the importance of listening to the chief complaint. But it is also important to listen beyond the chief complaint, to hear what isn't being said. That requires the use of all our senses. What is the patient's mood? What is the anxiety level? What is the body language telling us? Osler wisely counseled, "Listen to the patient. He is telling you the diagnosis."

Making a clinical diagnosis is akin to playing the popular game of twenty questions, in which the players attempt to guess the identity of the secret person. It is important to start broadly and selectively narrow the possibilities. In the game, for example, one might ask: Is it a man? Is he alive? Is he famous? And so on. Neurological disorders can be extremely complex, and I think it is prudent to simplify things whenever possible. When trying to make a diagnosis, there are always three questions I ask myself:

1. Is this a problem in the nervous system? (Or could it be a medical or psychiatric problem mimicking neurologic disease?)
2. If there is a neurological problem, can I localize it in the nervous system? (Does it involve the brain, spinal cord, or peripheral nerves? What structures and substructures could be involved, for example, the medial aspect of the dominant temporal lobe?)
3. What specific conditions could explain the patient's complaints? (For example, tumor, stroke, bleed, or inflammation.) Further diagnostic studies, including analysis of bloodwork, cerebrospinal fluid, electroencephalography, CT, MRI, and so on, can then help narrow the list of considerations.

Maybe that sounds like an oversimplification. But when trying to identify the cause of an illness, it is important to keep an open mind, start broadly so as not to go too far down the wrong path. Take Vinny's case, for example. One of the more common sites for brain tumors in children is the fourth ventricle, the location of Vinny's tumor. Vinny's tumor announced itself by causing balance difficulties. Often, tumors in this area cause vomiting, either by blocking the egress of CSF, leading to hydrocephalus and increased intracranial pressure, or by direct irritation of the brainstem. Sometimes tumors in the fourth ventricle activate the area postrema of the medulla oblongata at the lower brainstem, the so-called vomiting center, and kids may suffer from emesis, even to the point of weight loss.

If the tumor is largely within the CSF-filled fourth ventricle, it might not create other neurological abnormalities early on, such as weakness, sensory changes, or balance difficulties. For this reason, the correct diagnosis can be missed. Sometimes, kids with fourth ventricular brain tumors are sent to me after undergoing an extensive medical workup looking for gastrointestinal disease or a psychiatric workup looking for behavioral abnormalities. The physician who fails to consider the possibility of a neurologic cause for such complaints will fail to make the diagnosis.

When I finished examining Vinny, Rahul took him for a tour of the hospital. Priyanka stayed on, and I showed her the MRI and the location of the tumor. The top two diagnostic considerations were medulloblastoma and ependymoma. I'm sure that sounded like gibberish to her, but she had already read about these tumors and knew the bottom line. Both tumors are malignant. At that point, Priyanka broke down and wept. The whole ordeal with Vinny had happened so quickly that she hadn't had time to prepare herself.

Priyanka and Rahul were both born in New Delhi, India. Priyanka's grandfather was a math teacher in India who emigrated to the United States and subsequently brought members of his family here. Priyanka's father was a veterinarian in India, and her mother was an MBA student. Priyanka was born in New Delhi. She moved to New Jersey with her parents when she was twenty days old. Her father's veterinary degree was not accepted here, so he began pushing carts in a grocery store and ultimately was able to own several grocery stores in New York City. Her mother gave up her academic training to raise their kids.

Priyanka studied biology in college and thought about going to medical school but felt she didn't have the bandwidth to do that. She began working as a sales representative for a pharmaceutical company. Her romance with Rahul was orchestrated by her family, who heard about him through friends. They described him as a dashing young software developer in New Delhi. Priyanka's father traveled to India to meet him and look for other marital prospects for his young daughter. He was impressed by Rahul, and when he returned to New Jersey, he implored Priyanka to check him out.

Priyanka and Rahul corresponded for six months, sending messages to each other on AOL and using calling cards to talk. They hit it off immediately. She found him to be bright and caring, with a great sense of humor. He described himself to Priyanka as a great catch, the most eligible bachelor in town, with marriage requests from over fifty women. He told Priyanka to decide quickly before someone else snatched him away.

Priyanka was smitten. She flew to New Delhi in January 2009 to meet Rahul and instantly knew he was the right one. Her family flew over to New Delhi for their storybook arranged marriage a month later on Valentine's Day. She was twenty-four years old, and he was twenty-five. Rahul moved to New Jersey, where they are raising their two boys. He works as a senior software developer for vaccines and research for Pfizer, and Priyanka oversees a retail energy service company.

I sat with Priyanka and answered her questions. She composed herself and went over plans with me. Vinny would need a repeat MRI of his brain with intravenous gadolinium contrast to better define the tumor, along with an MRI of the entire spine, because sometimes fourth ventricular tumors can metastasize elsewhere in the nervous system. He would also need a wand

MRI of his brain to enable us to use frameless stereotactic image guidance in the OR to help us more precisely identify the margins of the tumor.

The hospital was bustling, and the OR schedule was full, but we were able to find a slot to do the MRI the following evening at one of our satellite facilities. The surgery would be performed the following morning on Thursday, February 17. Unfortunately, things didn't go as smoothly as planned.

Vinny and his family showed up for the MRI at 7 p.m., but the radiology team had a great deal of difficulty inserting an IV. Vinny was dehydrated, and his veins were small. He had never had any significant trouble with needles before, but it was the night before a big surgery, and he was frightened and became uncooperative.

We are usually prepared for things like this, with a pediatric anesthesia team available to provide sedation for the study. But the scan was set up urgently to enable us to operate the next morning, and there was no one from pediatrics and no one from anesthesia available to provide sedation. The radiology team called me, and I spoke to the family. We needed the contrast-enhanced MRI before surgery to show us the true extent and location of the tumor. We would have to cancel the surgery and bring Vinny back the following week for the sedated scan and surgery. Somehow, though, the family was able to calm Vinny down, and the scan was completed. It was a traumatic experience for all, but Vinny and his parents finally left to spend the night with relatives who lived nearby.

The family got up very early the next morning. Uncles, aunts, and cousins had come from around the country to wish them well. They started a "village prayer and chant session" that continued throughout the day, as Vinny and his parents left for the hospital.

I met them in the pre-op area at 5:30 a.m., and we went over plans and got consent for the surgery. Vinny brought along two stuffed animal sharks that he got when visiting the aquarium the previous day. One was named Jaws, and the other was Camo, because his scales were camouflaged. I promised that we would do the same operation on the sharks and have them recover together with Vinny in the ICU. Vinny was still shell-shocked from the night before. He stayed on his mom's lap and refused to get onto the hospital bed. He wouldn't put on his hospital gown. He was miserable.

Fortunately, an experienced and compassionate Child Life specialist handed him an iPad with a *Star Wars* game to distract him. And an experienced anesthesiologist gave him a liquid cocktail to calm him. That double-team combo worked so well that Vinny became laser-focused on the game and didn't even bother to say goodbye to his parents as he was whisked off to the OR.

With Vinny anesthetized on the OR table, we positioned him prone with his head slightly elevated and secured in a specialized holder. I was fortunate to have two exceptional assistants, Baha Muhsen and Tej Azad. We made a linear vertical incision in the midline at the back of Vinny's head, removed a trap-door portion of the skull, and opened the dura that protected the brain. Then, working under magnification provided by the operating microscope, we advanced our way toward the tumor, which was sitting on the right side of the fourth ventricle. To get there, we used a telovelar approach, dividing some fibrous membranes that allowed us to expose the tumor with minimal retraction of the cerebellum.

The tumor was soft, purplish, and very vascular. It bled profusely during the resection. We were able to control the bleeding with a bipolar coagulator and a variety of liquid hemostatic agents. It was a difficult case, but after several grueling hours, we were able to achieve a gross total resection. We then closed up and put Vinny back together. We gave him a cute head wrap and placed identical wraps on his stuffed animals, Jaws and Camo, so they could all recover together. I went to see Vinny's parents.

Priyanka and Rahul were in the waiting room along with Shivani and Ajay. Recalling the hours-long wait, Priyanka later told me she was a nervous wreck, and Rahul could barely speak. They were fearful of the unknown. Their minds were racing. Would their son wake up? Would he be paralyzed? Would he be a vegetable? Priyanka had bought a salad from the cafeteria but couldn't eat anything. She had lost ten pounds over the past few weeks. Rahul had lost more weight. Their perfect life had been shattered by Vinny's brain tumor.

"The operation went well," I said. "It's a small, round, blue cell tumor, which means it's malignant, a form of brain cancer. But we were able to remove everything we could see, and the brain looked good. The pathologists couldn't give us any further information at this time, but it looked like a medulloblastoma to us in the OR. It will take the pathologists several days to make the final diagnosis—they have to do a series of special stains and special studies. But Vinny's doing okay. He's been extubated—the breathing tube is out, and he's waking up nicely."

I brought mom and dad to see him in the ICU. I'm sure my description of what we called a medulloblastoma went in one ear for them and out the other. Most families, even those who are medically sophisticated, are so tense and apprehensive that they don't retain much of what is said. But they were relieved to see

Vinny and his sharks with their head wraps. Vinny had his eyes open and was sleepy but spoke to them. He had some weakness on the right side of his face, and his right arm was unsteady. But he looked better than they thought he would look. And I'm glad we fashioned head dressings for his fluffy pets, Jaws and Camo. It brought a smile to Vinny's face. Sometimes, some of the simplest things we do can have a lasting impact.

Vinny's facial weakness and unsteadiness continued to improve. He underwent intensive physical and occupational therapy in the hospital. His recovery was complicated by the development of a pseudomeningocele, an accumulation of cerebrospinal fluid under the scalp at the site of his surgical excision, which required placement of a temporary lumbar spinal drain to bring down the fluid collection.

It was a bumpy course, but Vinny's facial weakness ultimately resolved, as did his pseudomeningocele, and he recovered his neurological function.

The pathology returned as classic medulloblastoma, WHO grade 4. That's a high-grade embryonal (primitive) neoplasm, an aggressive form of brain cancer. That designation is based on microscopic analysis of the tumor's cellular architecture and mitoses (cellular divisions) with special staining. In the current era, we also analyze the tumor using next-generation sequencing (NGS), looking for unique mutations in the tumor that can potentially be targeted with novel drug therapies.

The pathologists performed a genetic analysis of Vinny's tumor and identified it as a Wingless Integrated Tumor (WNT) subtype. The designation WNT represents a combination of the terms Wingless and Integrated. The Wingless designation represents a cellular signaling pathway that was initially described by scientists decades ago in studies of *Drosophila melanogaster*, the common fruit fly. Vinny's WNT-activated medulloblastoma meant that it had mutations in *CTNNB1*, a gene that encodes a protein called beta-catenin. Beta-catenin accumulates in the nucleus of these tumor cells and propels tumorigenesis.

The medulloblastoma subtype terminology can sound pretty dense. But it conveys important information about prognosis. WNT-activated medulloblastoma is the least common subtype of these tumors, representing only 10 percent of the total. But WNT medulloblastomas are associated with the best overall prognosis, with a ten-year event-free survival rate of over 95 percent. Although medulloblastoma is a highly malignant brain cancer, we can now approach children with this tumor with the goal of achieving a cure. That's impressive because medulloblastoma was once considered a uniformly fatal tumor.

An interesting finding in WNT medulloblastomas is aberrant fenestrated blood vessels. This may explain why they can be so vascular at surgery. These blood vessel fenestrations cause a lack of a functional blood-brain barrier, which can enable improved access of chemotherapy to the tumor, thereby improving the prognosis of these tumors.

Armed with the favorable WNT diagnosis, we outlined a plan with our medical and radiation oncology colleagues to attempt to cure Vinny of his tumor.

The standard adjuvant (Latin for "to help") therapy for medulloblastoma is a combination of radiation and chemotherapy. Each of these modalities is toxic to the tumor but can also be toxic to the patient. Because of the encouraging WNT pathology, efforts are now underway to de-escalate the adjuvant therapy for this tumor subtype to reduce the associated side effects.

But there was a wrinkle in Vinny's case. Medulloblastoma is a malignant tumor that can metastasize throughout the nervous system. Before beginning adjuvant therapy, patients undergo an extensive disease workup that includes an MRI of the brain and entire spine, as well as a lumbar puncture (spinal tap). Vinny's brain MRI was clean after surgery, but his spine MRI showed that the tumor had metastasized lower down in the lumbosacral region inside the dura around the nerve roots. These were drop metastases, colloquially called drop mets. Spread to the spine was confirmed by the finding of tumor cells in the cerebrospinal fluid from the lumbar puncture.

The fact that Vinny's tumor had already metastasized was worrisome, but even so, it is possible to cure patients with the WNT-activated medulloblastoma subtype. And that's what we set out to do. What it meant for Vinny is that he would need to receive full-blown high-dose craniospinal radiation and multi-agent intravenous chemotherapy through an indwelling port placed through the skin into his superior vena cava.

Vinny was enrolled in a prospective high-risk medulloblastoma protocol by the Children's Oncology Group (COG) called ACNS 0332. He was randomized and assigned to a regimen to receive high-dose (fifty-four gray) proton beam radiation therapy to the brain and spinal cord, administered in thirty sessions over six weeks. A gray is a unit of the amount of radiation absorbed. Vinny had to be put to sleep for each session.

His chemotherapy consisted of an assortment of high-powered drugs, including vincristine, cyclophosphamide, and cisplatin, administered over a period of six months. Vincristine, as I described in an earlier chapter, is a plant-derived vinca alkaloid from the Madagascar periwinkle plant that blocks the growth of cells by interfering with microtubule polymerization. Cyclophosphamide is a synthetic alkylating agent derived in the 1950s from mustard gas. It causes cell death by impairing

DNA replication. It is also a potent immunosuppressive agent. Cisplatin is a heavy metal platinum-based alkylating agent that attacks DNA. Cisplatin was discovered by accident in 1965 and was approved by the FDA in 1978.

This was not an easy time for Vinny, who experienced multiple unpleasant side effects, including nausea, anorexia, fatigue, weight loss, high-frequency hearing loss, pancytopenia (low blood counts), and sepsis. He developed hydrocephalus (water on the brain) that required us to place a ventriculoperitoneal shunt to divert the excess cerebrospinal fluid to his abdomen, where it could be reabsorbed into his bloodstream.

Medulloblastoma accounts for about 20 percent of brain tumors in children and is the most common malignant brain tumor of childhood. More than two-thirds of medulloblastomas occur in children under the age of ten. The tumor was first described by the neurosurgeon Harvey Cushing and the neurosurgeon and neuropathologist Percival Bailey in 1925. They believed that it arose from a primitive multipotential embryonal cell called the medulloblast. It is interesting how the term medulloblastoma has survived the test of time, even though no multipotential medulloblast cell type has ever been identified. The term likely persisted because of the larger-than-life personality of its descriptor, Harvey Cushing, who founded the modern field of neurosurgery.

In recent years, there has been an explosion of research in the molecular biology of brain tumors. Medulloblastoma, which was considered for decades to be a single type of brain tumor, is now recognized to have multiple subtypes based on molecular genomic profiling. And now there are subtypes of the subtypes, with an alphabet soup of names that are difficult to remember, based on various genomic alterations, mutations, and amplifications. The hope, though, is that some of these molecular signatures can be targeted, leading to improvements in survival and mitigation of the side effects of treatment.

Even though Vinny came to us with a disseminated malignant central nervous neoplasm, the fact that it was a WNT-activated medulloblastoma gave those of us treating him a reason to hope for a cure. Throughout the course, Vinny remained stoic and helped his parents and older brother Veer navigate through these troubled waters. Once the treatments stopped, we could all see a light at the end of the tunnel. Over the next several months, Vinny's appetite returned, and he regained all the weight he had lost. His hair grew back. His sense of humor returned. His mediport catheter was removed. And his follow-up surveillance MRIs remained clean, with no evidence of tumor. We all breathed easier. Vinny got his childhood back.

In March 2023, a little over a year after Vinny's surgery, we noticed a very slight change in his follow-up cranial MRI. There was a new small shadow on the right side of his cerebellum adjacent to the site of his original tumor. It was only eight millimeters in maximal diameter and wasn't causing any irritation to the surrounding brain. But it showed enhancement after the administration of intravenous contrast, and it restricted diffusion. This caught our attention.

Could the tumor be coming back? There was no abnormality anywhere else in the brain or spinal cord. And Vinny was doing better clinically than he had ever been. We showed the film to all the experts at our weekly Tumor Board and debated what this meant. Was it a radiation-induced change? Or was it tumor recurrence? Sometimes radiation can create enhancing shadows on MRI that are not neoplastic and will ultimately go away. We didn't want to put Vinny through another surgery only to find that what we thought might be recurrent tumor was just an effect of the radiation. We chose to continue to follow Vinny with short-interval MRIs.

I was distressed to learn from Priyanka that one day, when Vinny awakened from a nap, he said, "Mama, I have a sense that I'm gonna pass away." Those are heartbreaking words to hear from anyone, particularly an eight-year-old boy. I called him to give him a pep talk. We had a video chat. He looked terrific. He told me about his new six-month-old puppy, Milo, a Maltese-poodle mix. He really loved the dog. I told him that I hoped Milo would be able to help him get through this next year of treatments. A loving pet is one of the best medicines around. Vinny told me that Milo was having some behavioral difficulties in doggy training school.

I told him about my dog Morty, a lovable 190-pound Newfoundland, who also had some behavior problems. I had wanted Morty to become a pet therapy dog at the hospital. But in order to do that, he had to go to Canine Good Citizenship School. Sadly, Morty failed the final exam on two counts. First, he had to walk across a room with treats scattered on the floor and not eat any of them. That was an immediate fail. Second, he decided to sniff the butt of the female trainer who gave the final exam. Fail again. I appealed to her, to no avail, that he was just being friendly. "Rules are rules," she said icily. So, I had to live with the humiliation that my loving dog Morty failed Canine Good Citizenship School. Instead, I had to sneak him into the hospital cafeteria from time to time so he could play with the kids. Vinny promised to keep me up to date about Milo's training.

Vinny remained perfectly well, but the contrast-enhancing diffusion-restricting shadow in his right cerebellum persisted on subsequent MRIs and got a little larger. That made our suspicion of recurrent tumor higher and of radiation change lower. So, we bit the bullet and made the difficult decision to reoperate on Vinny. On June 5, 2023, we went back to the OR. The operation was challenging because there was scar tissue from the prior operation and radiation that we had to work through. Fortunately, I had two superb assistants, Adam Ammar and Jawad Khalifeh, and we were able to localize the mass and remove it with clean margins. It was soft, reddish-gray, and vascular, but it didn't bleed as much as the tumor did at his first operation.

Vinny bounced back from this surgery much quicker than he did from the original resection. We were all disheartened to learn that the pathology was a recurrent tumor. Once again, it was a WNT-activated medulloblastoma, the identical pathology as it was at the time of his initial presentation. His post-op MRI looked clean once again, with no visible evidence of tumor.

Why did this tumor come back? What were we going to do now? It didn't make sense. The tumor wasn't behaving the way it was supposed to behave. WNT was the medulloblastoma subtype with the most favorable prognosis. All of the consultants met several times, informally and formally at our Tumor Board, to work out a plan. Statistics can only give us a certain amount of information. Medulloblastoma is indeed a malignant brain cancer, and even in our age of high technology, not everyone can be cured. But we were not about to throw in the towel.

Of the numerous molecular alterations in Vinny's tumor, one was a *TP53* gene mutation, which, according to some, but not all, studies might portend a more aggressive tumor. *TP53* stands for Tumor Protein 53. *TP53* is a tumor-suppressor gene that has also been called the "guardian of the genome" because of its function in regulating the cell cycle. Mutation of the *TP53* gene has a role in the development of several cancers, but its role in WNT medulloblastoma is less clear.

I suspect all of us—the family and the physicians—were in a bit of denial during the weeks leading up to the reoperation. But we knew we had to act. And we worked with local and national experts and decided to treat Vinny with a new COG protocol, ACNS 0821. This time, he would receive a lower dose (thirty-five gray) of proton beam radiation directed at the tumor bed over a period of ten days. This time, his multi-agent chemotherapy would consist of temozolomide (an alkylating agent that damages DNA) along with bevacizumab (an angiogenesis inhibitor that blocks the growth of blood vessels) and irinotecan (a topoisomerase inhibitor that blocks an enzyme that plays a role in DNA replication). The goal was to triple team the effort and target different drivers of tumor growth. A big hit for a little guy.

Vinny finished his course of focused proton radiation therapy without a problem. He finally completed his second round of adjuvant chemotherapy. The tumor and the treatments took a toll. It was hard for him to see a light at the end of the tunnel when he was indoors recovering from the toxicities of treatment, while his classmates were outside playing soccer and baseball and football. On a surveillance MRI performed three months after Vinny's second surgery, there were small shadows in the area of the tumor resection. This raised concern that they might represent tumor recurrence. Fortunately, these shadows disappeared on a repeat MRI performed after another three months. His most recent MRI, done one year after his second surgery, showed no evidence of tumor recurrence.

Vinny has the strength of a superhero. He bounced back after completing his radiation and chemotherapy. He finished third grade without a problem. He's eating like a horse and gaining weight back. He's now eleven years old and doing very well in school in the fifth grade. He's a bundle of energy, running, swimming, and playing with friends, making up for lost time. He told me he swam twelve laps in his grandparents' pool over the weekend. He likes to play pickleball with his brother Veer. But he gets tired quickly and still has to rest a lot. He plays a lot of video games and does puzzles on his iPad.

Thanks to the Make-A-Wish Foundation, one of Vinny's lifelong dreams has come true. This summer, he went to California to work as a zookeeper at the San Diego Zoo and Sea World. I thought it was a bizarre wish. He told me it was on his list of key things he needed to do in life. He wants to save the sea turtles and sea otters as well as the rhinoceroses. I was impressed and told Vinny that I thought he'd made a very noble choice. Most kids want to take an expensive vacation or go to Disney World. He's the only eleven-year-old I know who wants to be a zookeeper. I asked him if he was certain he didn't want to go to Disney World.

"Oh, absolutely certain," he said. "I've really got to save the animals. I did a school project this year on endangered species, and things look really bad for the sea turtles. They need me. The burden is on my shoulders. But I won't be able to make a living as a zookeeper alone. I'm planning to moonlight as a brain surgeon."

Vinny is an incredible kid, truly one of a kind, who marches to his own beat. He is filled with hope in his heart, and all of us on his medical team stand behind him. We celebrate his remission from brain cancer, and we hold our breath. We don't know what the future holds, but we are guided by the combination of technology and optimism. That's the roller coaster we ride.

Even when things look bleak, it's essential to hang on to hope. Vinny has a loving family and a team of doctors and nurses doing their best to help him through this terrible ordeal. It's important for him to have the right mindset, to keep fighting, to stay optimistic. And it is equally important for the treating physicians to share that hope. There is a healing power of optimism. It's impossible to care for children with brain tumors without having a positive outlook. Being optimistic doesn't mean ignoring the reality of the circumstances. It means maintaining hope, even in the face of adversity.

Or in the words of Theodore Roosevelt, "When you're at the end of your rope, tie a knot and hold on."

CHAPTER 14
Revelation

"It is unwise to be too sure of one's own wisdom. It is healthy to be reminded that the strongest might weaken and the wisest might err."

MAHATMA GANDHI
FEBRUARY 17, 1940
HARIJAN ("CHILDREN OF GOD"),
GANDHI'S WEEKLY NEWSPAPER

Tuesday, April 8, 2008, began uneventfully for Jackie and Todd Bertolette. It was unseasonably warm, moderately cloudy, and a light rain was falling. They were taking their newborn son, Trent, for a routine checkup with Dr. Diane Lester, his pediatrician in Mentor, Ohio. Trent was a healthy ten-week-old infant boy who was born on January 27 at thirty-nine weeks' gestation via normal spontaneous vaginal delivery. Jackie's pregnancy was uncomplicated. Trent's birthweight was eight pounds, eight ounces. He was feeding well at home and gaining weight, with no health concerns. He had two older siblings: Sebastian, age eight, and Skylar, age six, who were both healthy.

The visit began with a routine check of Trent's vital signs by the nurse and a customary physical exam by the doctor. All findings were normal until the final, seemingly harmless measurement, Trent's occipitofrontal head circumference. His head was large, measuring forty-four centimeters, greater than the 97th percentile. That came as a bit of a surprise. But he looked so good. Why should his head be so large? Newborn babies are often squirrelly and don't like to hold still, which can sometimes lead to a measurement error. Dr. Lester checked again and asked several nurses to come in and take another reading. All measurements were the same—Trent had an enlarged head, a condition called macrocephaly (Greek: *makros*, "large," *kephale*, "head"). The only other finding on his exam was that his anterior fontanelle, the soft spot on top of the head in the midline, was a little full, a finding that can also be a variation of normal.

Macrocephaly itself is not necessarily a concern. Some kids have big heads; some kids have small heads. With newborns and infants, measurement error is common. Macrocephaly can be a concern if a single measurement of the head circumference is greater than two standard deviations above the mean, or if the head circumference crosses percentiles on serial measurements. There are three general causes for true congenital macrocephaly: enlargement of the brain itself (macrencephaly), enlargement of the CSF spaces (e.g., hydrocephalus), or the presence or enlargement of other structures (e.g., brain tumor, or intracranial hematoma).

Macrocephaly is a relatively common finding during a well-child examination by the pediatrician. One of the most common causes is benign enlargement of the subarachnoid space (BESS), in which there is a little extra CSF over the convexities of the brain. It is a mild self-limited form of hydrocephalus that does not require treatment and runs its course over the first two years of life. A variant of BESS is familial macrocephaly, a relatively common condition, in which big heads run in the family without causing any harm. Curiously, Trent's father, Todd, did have a big head.

Dr. Lester was deliberating about what to do. Confronted with a healthy child like Trent during a well-child visit, most pediatricians would send the family home and bring the kid back for serial measurements of the head circumference. Trent's head circumference was only slightly above what was acceptable. Dr. Lester told Jackie and Todd that she was going back and forth in her mind about whether to send Trent for a CT scan of his head. Finally, she said she would rather err on the side of caution, and she scheduled an immediate CT.

So, Todd went home to wait for the two older kids to return from school. And Jackie, still unconcerned, took Trent down the hall to Radiology for the scan. When Trent was in the scanner for over an hour, Jackie began to feel apprehensive. She became more alarmed, and her heart began to pound when she saw the look on Dr. Lester's face. Dr. Lester told Jackie the scan showed a massive tumor involving the entire right hemisphere of Trent's brain. Dr. Lester was solemn. She had never had to deliver this kind of news before. She would send Trent immediately by ambulance to see us in the ER at Rainbow Babies and Children's Hospital for further evaluation.

Jackie was numb. She began to realize the gravity of the situation when the staff got her coffee, brought her a chair, and offered her the use of the phone. She was rattled and began to sob when the radiology technician approached her and embraced her, explaining how sorry she was. She gave Jackie hard copies of the CT to bring along to the hospital.

Jackie felt as if time had frozen during the thirty-minute ambulance ride to the hospital. She sat in the back with Trent, consumed with fear. She had recently lost her aunt to a brain tumor. Now this. The paramedic sitting with them stared blankly and silently at the scans. Todd rushed to the hospital to meet them in the ER.

The Bertolettes were greeted by the ER triage team, who examined Trent and had him admitted to the pediatric intensive care unit (PICU). Trent was sedated and whisked off for a two-hour MRI of his brain to better delineate the nature of the large mass in his right hemisphere. At 9:30 p.m., eight hours after Trent had arrived at his routine well-child visit with the pediatrician, I met with his parents to deliver the news about his giant malignant brain tumor.

I had already reviewed the MRI with the attending neuroradiologist and other members of our neurosurgical team. There was a large enhancing cystic and solid multi-lobulated mass filling the right hemisphere of the brain, spilling over to the left side, resulting in significant brain compression. There was cerebral edema (swelling), causing a shift of the brain from right to left. Sometimes brain tumors can spread to other sites across the nervous system, which is why we also performed an MRI of the spine. Fortunately, the spine was normal.

Jackie, who was a very strong woman, took one look at the MRI and collapsed backward into her husband's arms. We got her settled down, and I began the difficult task of explaining that Trent had a life-threatening problem that we would address expeditiously with surgery scheduled for 6 a.m. the following morning. The prognosis was grave. The purpose of surgery was to make a tissue diagnosis to determine the exact nature of the brain tumor and to remove as much of it as was safely possible.

Later on, Jackie reminded me that after going through all the sobering details for the surgical informed consent, I said, trying to muster a sense of confidence, "Don't worry, we have a good plan. I got this."

I'm not sure if that helped to calm the family down. But they did request to meet with the hospital chaplain, a wonderful woman whom they felt was very comforting and helpful.

We operated on Trent the next morning at the crack of dawn. Jackie remembers "being in a strange dreamlike state as I watched a slew of medical personnel calmly wheel my ten-week-old angel to the OR, attached to a series of portable monitors and IVs." Friends and family had made their way to the hospital to provide moral support during the agonizing hours in the waiting room while the surgery was being carried out. Jackie was despondent and kept poring over the pregnancy and delivery, wondering if there was something she had done wrong to cause Trent's fate.

I performed the operation with Shakeel Chowdhry, an exceptionally bright senior neurosurgery resident. After Trent was asleep under general endotracheal anesthesia, we placed a bump under his right shoulder and positioned his head parallel to the floor on a padded horseshoe rest. Before coming to the OR, we had marked the right side of Trent's head and confirmed the site of surgery during a time-out performed in the OR.

The time-out is a routine maneuver we perform in every case to make certain that the entire team is on the same page. We run through a checklist much the same as airline pilots do in the cockpit before takeoff. While brain surgery can be complex, it's often the simple things that can go wrong and cause a misadventure in the OR. Like operating on the wrong side of the head. Which is why we always mark the surgical site preoperatively and double-check it in the OR before starting the case.

We shaved Trent's head and outlined a large question mark incision with the inferior limb just in front of the tragus, the tongue-like external projection of his right ear, and the medial limb directly on the midline. The scalp is very vascular, which is one of the reasons it heals so well. To reduce bleeding, we injected the scalp with a dilute solution containing epinephrine, and we used sterile plastic Raney clips to compress the edges of the incision. This is particularly important in young kids because their blood volume is small, and they don't have that much blood to lose. Then we used a power saw to elevate a large craniotomy, which consisted of a fronto-temporo-parieto-occipital bone flap. Essentially, we exposed the entire right side of his brain. Fashioning the craniotomy was easy. We didn't even need to make burr holes because the soft spot, his anterior fontanelle, was wide open from underlying increased intracranial pressure. The skull was so thin that we were able to remove a good portion of it using scissors.

Once we removed the bone flap and opened the fibrous dura mater covering the brain, the first thing we noticed was a horrible rancid odor that permeated the room and smelled like a large batch of rotten eggs. I instantly knew the correct diagnosis. We looked closer at the surface of the brain under magnification of the operating microscope and saw an astonishing sight. The surface of the brain was covered by a thick yellow creamy substance, with large pockets of purulent material inside the brain as well. It was pus. There was no tumor at all. Trent had bacterial meningitis that had spread inside the brain in a series of loculated pockets as brain abscesses filling the entire right hemisphere.

We drained the pus on the cerebral surface and opened the brain in multiple sites, evacuating a huge amount of pus from the abscesses. We sent this material off to the microbiology lab for cultures, irrigated the brain with antibiotic solution, closed the dura, replaced the bone flap, and sutured the scalp. The brain, which was under high pressure when we opened, was now soft and relaxed, much more normal.

We were relaxed too. What looked like a highly malignant brain tumor wasn't a tumor at all. It was a bacterial infection. And although it was a substantial and atypical infection, a brain abscess, unlike most malignant brain tumors, can be treated and cured. The anesthesia team extubated Trent, and I scurried off to the waiting room to tell the family the good news.

"When we exposed the brain," I said, smiling broadly, "the first thing we noted was a god-awful smell."

My excitement was not shared by the family. They were flabbergasted. I had finished the operation hours earlier than they expected it would take for resection of a malignant brain tumor. Why did we finish so much earlier than they expected? Had something gone wrong in the OR? Was the tumor inoperable? Had I lost my mind? How could I speak so flippantly about their precious, adorable infant son, who was the picture of health just twenty-four hours ago and then taken away to the OR earlier in the day at death's door?

I sensed the tension in the room and immediately clarified my message. That god-awful smell was the best news I could bring them. Brain tumors don't usually smell. Trent did not have brain cancer. It was an infection. A brain abscess. Their child was not going to die. Mom and dad looked at each other and then at me. The tension broke. Tears of happiness filled the room. Then hugs. Then laughter. It was the first time since the saga began that they had laughed.

The next several days were stressful. Trent was monitored in the PICU. He had several generalized seizures caused by irritation of the cerebral cortex from the infection. We treated him with broad-spectrum antibiotics and anti-seizure medication. Since he would need long-term antibiotics, we placed a peripherally inserted central catheter (PICC), a thin, flexible tube that went into a vein in his arm and was threaded centrally to end in a larger vein, the superior vena cava.

Cultures from the OR grew *Citrobacter koseri*. The bacterium *Citrobacter* was first identified in 1932. *Citrobacter koseri* is a gram-negative non-spore-forming facultative anaerobic bacillus. That means it is a rod-shaped organism that grows in the absence of oxygen, anaerobically, but is capable of growing aerobically, in the presence of oxygen. It is found in soil and water and is part of the normal flora of the human gastrointestinal tract.

Citrobacter koseri is a rare but particularly devastating cause of neonatal meningitis and brain abscess. The reason Trent developed a fulminant *Citrobacter* brain infection was not clear. He was treated with a combination of surgery and a prolonged course of two powerful intravenous antibiotics, gentamicin and meropenem. Because brain abscesses are walled-off infections, surgery is required to drain the purulent collections and allow the antibiotics to penetrate the site of infection.

Trent started to improve slowly. An MRI done one week after surgery showed that the brain looked significantly better, with a marked reduction in the abscess load. But there was one large, round, deep-seated, walled-off abscess that had not been drained. So Shakeel and I went back to the OR with Trent and performed an MRI-guided frameless stereotactic aspiration of that pocket of residual pus. We were able to do that by using a special MRI sequence that allowed us to translate the two-dimensional anatomy of the MRI into the three-dimensional anatomy of the OR, essentially creating a GPS for the brain. This allowed us to track our instruments and place a catheter into the deep abscess with pinpoint precision and drain the residual pus through a small burr hole.

Trent continued to make gains, but a week later, he had another generalized seizure, despite being on anti-seizure medication. We repeated an MRI and an MR venogram (MRV), which showed a thrombus (blood clot) in the right transverse sinus, a large vein that drains blood from the brain back to the heart. This likely occurred because of the irritative effects of the extensive intracranial infection, which made Trent hypercoagulable. If untreated, venous sinus thrombosis can cause cerebral infarction, or stroke.

We treated him by continuing the antibiotics for weeks and weeks and adding a blood thinner. Dr. Nancy Bass of pediatric neurology did a beautiful job managing his seizures with levetiracetam and phenobarbital and overseeing his long-term care. Trent had spent five weeks in the PICU and continued to make slow but steady progress over several painstaking months. Jackie went to classes to learn how to manage the central line and got "certified" by the hospital staff. Under Jackie's watchful eye, Trent completed the final weeks of his antibiotics at home.

There were still several ups and downs. Trent remained lethargic during his first few weeks at home. We were not sure how much improvement he would ultimately achieve. The antibiotics had to be administered three times a day, and Jackie felt as if she had turned her living room into a hospital ICU. A home nurse came regularly to check on the antibiotic regimen and draw bloodwork to monitor the infection. In total, Trent received sixteen weeks of IV antibiotics, the majority of which were given by Jackie in her newfound role as a medical paraprofessional.

At one point, Trent developed severe diarrhea and colitis and had to be hospitalized again for a Clostridioides difficile (C. diff) infection of the large intestine. C. diff is a gram-positive spore-forming bacterial infection caused by immunosuppression in the setting of long-term antibiotic therapy. It is a serious problem, responsible for causing about half a million infections yearly in the United States. Trent had to be quarantined for a period in his hospital room and have his antibiotics changed until he recovered.

Finally, after several months at home, Trent turned the corner. He became more alert and went on to make a dramatic recovery. His MRIs showed resolution of the multifocal brain abscesses. With physical, occupational, and speech therapy, he regained the developmental milestones he had lost. He was able to rewire his brain and began to excel at things he was never expected to do. He continued his anti-seizure medications for two years and then stopped them, with no further seizures for six years. Subsequently, he has experienced occasional focal seizures involving only his jaw, which have been controlled with oxcarbazepine (Trileptal), another anti-seizure medication.

Recently, I met up with Trent and didn't recognize him. He is now eighteen years old with a full head of hair, and there's no hint that he had the entire right side of his skull removed and replaced to evacuate his multifocal brain abscess when he was a newborn baby. He's a typical, normal teenager, functioning well as an honor roll student in school. He's dyed his hair bright red. He walks, runs, jumps, and is a bundle of energy. He loves music and has become an accomplished drummer. He spends more time playing video games than Jackie would prefer.

His professional goal is to develop and market novel video games, although he has given some thought to becoming a professional drummer. His teacher, Mrs. Leon, and his classmates enjoy his weekly drum solos that he records on YouTube. He does volunteer work at a local art commune, and he and his family occasionally bring gift baskets to the PICU, where he spent the early portion of his life. His mother, Jackie, is an accomplished fashion editor and photographer as well as a couture designer, and his father, Todd, works as a lab technician at a steel mill.

Trent's saga is remarkable for several reasons. What appeared to be a malignant brain tumor to the entire medical team ended up being an infection, not any type of tumor at all. It's rare that we consider it to be good news when we tell a family that their young child has a giant, multilobulated brain abscess. But everything is relative. The reason we considered this good news is that a brain abscess is much more amenable to treatment than most brain cancers.

The treatment for a brain abscess is a combination of surgery and antibiotics, along with meticulous management of the potential complications along the way—for example, seizures, venous sinus thromboses, superinfections, and so on. For Trent, his care was delivered by a large team of specialists, including neurosurgeons, neurologists, intensivists, anesthesiologists, and infectious disease experts. In all, the team consisted of over twenty-five physicians and twenty nurses. Fortunately, in Trent's case, the treatment worked.

That is not to say, however, that Trent's multiloculated holohemispheric (entire side of the brain) *Citrobacter* abscess is something to be taken lightly. It was a serious, potentially lethal illness.

A cerebral abscess is a walled-off localized collection of pus in the brain caused by a bacterial or fungal infection. It is a disease of the young, with almost half of all reported brain abscesses occurring in children under the age of fifteen years. Most published series of brain abscesses document a two-to-one predominance of boys compared to girls. The classic presentation of a patient with a brain abscess is a triad of fever, headache, and focal neurological deficit. However, Trent had none of these findings, which made his diagnosis difficult. In fact, that classic triad is present in fewer than half the cases.

In newborns, the most common cause of a brain abscess is neonatal meningitis, an infection of the coverings of the brain. Trent's brain abscess was associated with meningitis caused by the bacterium *Citrobacter koseri*. *Citrobacter koseri* is a rare but very serious cause of neonatal meningitis and abscess. The more common organisms implicated are *Group B streptococcus*, *Escherichia coli*, and *Listeria monocytogenes*. Trent's *Citrobacter* meningitis and brain abscess were also associated with cerebral edema (brain swelling) and necrotizing meningoencephalitis (a dangerous inflammation of the brain and its coverings). These factors contribute to the unique dangers of neonatal *Citrobacter* brain infections.

The *Citrobacter* bacterium gets its name because the organism uses citrate as the sole source of carbon. Citrate, or citric acid, is a colorless organic acid occurring in the cell cycle that's created by the fermentation of sugars. It has a sour taste and is found in fruits such as lemons and limes.

Trent's *Citrobacter* brain infection was not a walk in the park by any means. Thirty percent of neonates with *Citrobacter* meningitis will die, and 50 percent will have a poor neurologic outcome. Three-fourths of all neonates with *Citrobacter koseri* meningitis will develop brain abscesses, as was the case with Trent.

And, as we found with Trent, *Citrobacter koseri* brain abscesses tend to be large and multifocal, making them difficult to treat.

Effective therapy consists of a combination of surgery and intravenous antimicrobial medication. Refractory abscesses may require further surgical drainage, as the antibiotics may not penetrate the thick capsule surrounding the purulent infection. We had to go back to the OR once with Trent. Some abscesses require multiple drainage procedures.

Jackie's pregnancy with Trent was uncomplicated, and Trent's birth was straightforward. Why, then, did he develop this near-fatal brain infection? The *Citrobacter* abscess can be caused by vertical transmission from the mother or horizontal transmission from the postnatal environment. In Trent's case, Jackie was completely healthy, and no cause for the infection could be identified. In fact, no cause is identified in most neonatal cases of *Citrobacter* brain abscess. Affected infants tend to be normal and lack other predisposing factors for brain abscess, including prematurity, low birth weight, fetal hypoxia, traumatic delivery, premature rupture of membranes (PROM), and an immunocompromised state.

Although it has been many years since I cared for Trent, I think about him frequently, for two reasons. The first is to remember that although *Citrobacter* brain abscess is a rare and exceedingly treacherous condition for which the cause is often not found, an aggressive combination of surgical and medical treatment can lead to a favorable outcome, even in fulminant cases. The second is more humbling. Why didn't I recognize the diagnosis until the time of surgery? In this age of high-tech neuroimaging and other diagnostic tools, how come the entire team caring for Trent mistook an infection for a malignant brain tumor?

This brings me back to Gandhi's words at the beginning of the chapter: "It is unwise to be too sure of one's own wisdom."

With all the extraordinary technology available to us, technology is merely a tool and can sometimes lead us down the wrong path. The MRI finding of large ring-enhancing diffusion-restricting masses filling the right hemisphere of Trent's brain was highly suggestive, but not pathognomonic, of a malignant tumor. There is only so much information that we can glean from our tools. Infection can be mimicked by other conditions on neuroimaging studies. What made Trent's case particularly difficult was the absence of findings on physical exam. We had actually considered brain abscess in the differential diagnosis of Trent's condition when we first saw the MRI; it was just lower down on the list.

Luckily, we would not have done anything different, even if a brain abscess was first on our list of potential diagnoses. For those of us in the medical profession, it is important to keep an open mind and not become too dogmatic in our thinking. While it is essential for the physician to develop a sense of self-confidence, we need to remember that many of the decisions we make are based on uncertainty.

I am frequently reminded of the words of Sir William Osler, "Medicine is a science of uncertainty and an art of probability." Things that are crystal clear in retrospect can be confusing in real time without the benefit of hindsight. In medicine, we often must make decisions about management before all the details are available.

One of the worst things a doctor can do is to become overconfident and intransigent in his or her way of thinking. I was fortunate to learn humility early in my neurosurgical training under the mentorship of Joseph Ransohoff, a world-class neurosurgeon. He was a demanding, hard-driving, chain-smoking, intrepid pioneer who sported a tattoo of a battleship on his arm.

But he was also a very wise man who had little tolerance for arrogance and conceit.

In our weekly neurosurgery clinical conferences, the other residents and I would often present difficult cases we had recently cared for, proudly showing the post-op MRI with no evidence of residual brain tumor. Ransohoff would never let us get cocky, though, always taking us down a notch and reminding us to maintain a modest view of our own importance. In fact, the plaque that hangs on my wall, which was given to me when I finished my neurosurgery residency training, is inscribed with the Latin phrase, "Melior fortunas quam bonus esse." It was our department's motto, chosen by Ransohoff himself. "Better to be lucky than good."

CHAPTER 15

Serendipity

"Serendipity. Look for something, find something else, and realize that what you've found is more suited to your needs than what you thought you were looking for."

Lawrence Block
American crime writer

For Carter Paxton, the day began unremarkably. It was mid-July in 2019, and he got up at about 7 a.m., had breakfast, and set out to do his daily chores, which included vacuuming the house, washing the dishes, and taking out the trash. Then he went to his room and read for a while before going online on his PlayStation 4 gaming console to play Minecraft and Fortnite with several of his friends. Later in the morning, his mother, Tobi, saw him and noticed that he looked pale.

"What's wrong?" she asked him. "You look sick. Are you feeling okay?"

"I don't know, Mom. I have a stomachache," he said. "I'm a little nauseous, and I have diarrhea. I don't feel so great. The same thing happened to me yesterday morning."

"Could it be something you ate?" she asked. "What did you have for breakfast?"

"Nothing special," he said. "Just some Cinnamon Toast Crunch."

Tobi went to the refrigerator and opened the carton of milk. "Oh my God, Carter!" she gasped. "This milk is spoiled. It smells awful. Why did you use it? Didn't it smell bad to you?"

"Mom, remember, I can't smell," he said.

Tobi felt terrible. She'd forgotten that her otherwise healthy twelve-year-old son had no sense of smell. He was unable to smell things as far back as she could remember. But it was never a real issue. Until now.

"I'm so sorry, Carter," she said. "I forgot. I hope you don't have a stomach infection. I'm taking you to see the doctor."

The Paxtons' family practitioner examined Carter and thought he had a mild case of gastroenteritis but looked pretty good overall. He had some concern about the profound, longstanding anosmia (loss of the sense of smell) and referred Carter to see an otolaryngologist, Dr. Nancy Solowski. They got an appointment to see her a few days later.

Dr. Solowski thought Carter might have a paranasal sinus infection and prescribed a two-week course of amoxicillin. Carter completed the antibiotic regimen and returned to see Dr. Solowski on August 14. There was no longer any evidence of infection, but Carter still couldn't smell a thing. Dr. Solowski confirmed this by giving him an olfactory test, which he promptly failed. She presented him with forty different substances to smell. His score was 0/40.

Dr. Solowski alerted the family that often, the cause of long-standing anosmia can remain elusive. Some general sources of anosmia include infection, nasal obstruction, and head trauma. Dr. Solowski was able to rule these out. During the COVID-19 pandemic, anosmia received a great deal of attention. In the setting of COVID-19, the loss of smell is usually transient, lasting a few weeks. The mechanism for anosmia in COVID-19 appears to be an immunologic reaction to the presence of the virus that transiently changes the architecture of the olfactory neurons in the nose.

Dr. Solowski felt Carter likely had congenital anosmia. Congenital anosmia is present at birth and can sometimes be associated with genetic syndromes. Carter didn't have a genetic syndrome, but his loss of smell dated back as far as he could remember. Kids with congenital anosmia may not realize they can't smell for several years of their early life. That was surely the case for Carter.

"I'm not completely sure why Carter can't smell," Dr. Solowski said. "So, I'm going to order an MRI of his brain. I want to get a good look at his olfactory system."

The MRI was performed at a regional imaging center on August 23, and Carter and his mother went to see Dr. Solowski in follow-up on September 4. Dr. Solowski reviewed the MRI with them. There was no abnormality involving the olfactory system, but the study was not normal. There was a mass in the right frontal lobe of Carter's brain. It had the appearance of a glioma, an intrinsic primary brain tumor, a tumor arising from the substance of the brain itself. Tobi began to cry. She wasn't prepared for this at all. Her mind started racing. She thought the MRI was going to be normal and was shocked to see the lesion in the right frontal lobe. She thought about brain surgery. About the risks of brain surgery. About the possibility of brain damage, even death. She didn't want Carter to see her. Carter began to cry, too, but didn't really know what any of this meant.

Dr. Solowski said, "I'm going to refer Carter to Dr. Alan Cohen, a friend of mine. He's a pediatric neurosurgeon. His patients call him 'Big Al.' I'll give him a call." At that point, Tobi went into a free fall. Her child had a temporary illness from drinking sour milk, and now there was talk of possible brain surgery.

Dr. Solowski was an experienced ENT surgeon who was also kind and compassionate. She showed Carter the scar on her own head from the brain tumor surgery she had undergone when she was a teenager. It was a moving gesture, and it helped to relax the tension in the room. She had undergone brain surgery, and she was perfectly normal. Coincidentally, her neurosurgeon so many years ago was Richard Fraser, the chief of neurosurgery at the New York Hospital/Cornell Medical Center. That's where I trained in medical school, and he was one of my teachers. Brilliant man. Small world.

Tobi and Carter got to the car, and both sat there and cried for several minutes. They turned on one of Carter's favorite playlists to listen to as they drove home.

I called the family and set up an appointment to see Carter that week. I saw and examined him in the clinic with our physician assistant, Heather Kerber. Aside from his lack of sense of smell, he was a perfectly healthy left-handed twelve-year-old boy. I showed the family the MRI and pointed out the bright white spot and the surrounding dark halo, representing the enhancing expansile mass in the right middle frontal gyrus (ridge-like elevation on the cerebral cortex) of Carter's brain and the surrounding edema. The mass measured 3.5 centimeters in diameter. We and the neuroradiologists who interpreted the scan felt it had the appearance of a low-grade glioma, a tumor arising from the gluelike glial supporting cells of the brain, with a small amount of surrounding brain swelling. The differential diagnosis also included other neoplasms, such as a dysembryoplastic neuroepithelial tumor (DNET) or a pleomorphic xanthoastrocytoma. Each of these is a low-grade tumor. But despite the great accuracy of MRI, there was no way to make the diagnosis without further intervention.

I recommended surgery to diagnose the lesion and remove it. Carter was left-handed. Most people are right-handed, and the language area is in their dominant cerebral hemisphere, on the left side of the brain. Most left-handed people also have their language center in the left hemisphere, but some may have it in the right hemisphere or even in both hemispheres. I was also concerned that the mass abutted the right motor cortex, the part of the brain responsible for voluntary movement of the left side of the body. In fact, there was one place where the mass invaded the motor cortex, the area responsible for movement of the left side of Carter's face.

Because we were concerned about the possible proximity of the mass to Carter's language area and its clear proximity to the motor cortex, we recommended a functional MRI (fMRI). The fMRI is a noninvasive test that can be useful in planning surgery by demonstrating the relationship of the lesion to critical brain structures. In an fMRI, the patient is asked to perform various tasks while the brain is being imaged on the scanner. The technique detects blood oxygen level dependent (BOLD) changes as a surrogate for neuronal activity, in this case helping to determine the location of language and motor function. fMRI is used infrequently in pediatric patients because it requires the cooperation of the child.

But Carter was a mature twelve-year-old who cooperated perfectly, and we were able to perform the fMRI on September 24, 2019. It showed that Carter's language center was largely in the left hemisphere of his brain, but there was some language function along the superior aspect of the lesion on the right side. It also confirmed the proximity of the right hemisphere mass to the motor fibers innervating the left side of Carter's face. This MRI study also included diffusion tensor imaging (DTI), a technique that analyzes the movement of water molecules down axons, the fibers that carry nerve impulses away from the nerve cell bodies. DTI can help identify the exact location of important white matter tracts (nerve fibers) in the brain. The fMRI/DTI study was a big help—it let us know exactly where we would need to be extra careful during the operation.

The Paxtons were a delightful family living in Odenton, Maryland, a charming town with a population of about twenty thousand located twenty miles from Baltimore and fifteen miles from Annapolis, the state capital. Tobi worked as a compliance and risk management advisor for Wells Fargo. Her husband, Richard, was a Navy man who worked at Fort Meade as a staff commander, advising officers and admirals about defensive measures for the country. He currently works for Deloitte and Touche as a cybersecurity expert. Their twelve-year-old son, Carter, was in the seventh grade. Carter's brother Lucas was two years older. Both were bright kids who were homeschooled.

Years later, Carter would tell me how it felt to learn as a twelve-year-old boy that he would need to have brain surgery to remove a tumor. "I went into the bathroom and sat there for at least twenty minutes, trying to calm down," he said. "My heart was pounding. My body was shaking. I felt like I was going to vomit. Finally, I came out of the bathroom and asked some questions about the surgery. The three things I was freaking out about were: using the sleeping gas to put me to sleep, getting my head cut open, and me being bald. That night, when I got home, I hid in the bathroom, texting my friends that this might be the last time they ever hear from me." Those are some somber thoughts for anyone, particularly a young, impressionable twelve-year-old.

We scheduled surgery for Monday, September 30, 2019. Carter's anxiety level was high. He had decided to give his brain tumor a name. He called it Carl. It was a name he had chosen at random. "I knew I had something in my head," he said. "I didn't really know what a brain tumor was, but it sounded scary. Calling it Carl seemed more comforting." That made perfect sense to me. In fact, Carter was not the only patient of mine who gave his tumor a name. I think it serves to help kids manage a frightening experience on their own terms.

Carter and his family met with a child life specialist during the week. She showed them the lay of the land in the hospital, including the pre-op area and the PICU where his parents could stay with him after the surgery. Carter's parents shaved his entire head on Friday night in preparation for the operation on Monday. He had a Wand MRI performed on Saturday. The study was done with the placement of temporary stickers on his head to help us localize the tumor when he would be asleep on the OR table. Later that Saturday, hoping to distract him, Carter's parents took him to play miniature golf and then to his favorite Mexican restaurant for a meal. The day before surgery, Carter went with his family to the mall, where they visited Bath and Body Works. He had a final reminder of his anosmia when he held the candles to his nose and had to ask his mother what they smelled like.

Monday was an early start, and Carter and his family were in the hospital at 5:30 a.m., well before sunrise. We had enrolled Carter in a voluntary national clinical trial assessing the efficacy of a novel agent for fluorescence-guided surgery for brain tumors. Our medical center was part of the study, which was conducted by the Pacific Pediatric Neuro-Oncology Consortium (PNOC). The study, PNOC-012, was a randomized, blinded investigation of fluorescence detection of pediatric primary central nervous system tumors in children receiving the intravenous agent, tozuleristide (also called "Tumor Paint"). The study was designed to investigate the role of tozuleristide administered preoperatively as a means of improving the resection of pediatric brain tumors by lighting up the tumors but not the brain.

Fluorescence-guided surgery is of interest to neurosurgeons because the removal of primary brain tumors can sometimes be difficult and tricky. These tumors arise from the substance of the brain itself and often don't have a capsule to delineate them from the normal surrounding tissue. Therefore, in certain cases, it can be difficult to determine where the tumor ends and the brain begins, even with the magnification provided by the operating microscope. Fluorescence-guided surgery is based on the principle that certain peptide compounds can bind to structures that are present in brain tumors but not in a normal brain.

Tozuleristide is a bioconjugate drug that contains a synthetic form of chlorotoxin bound to a derivative of the near-infrared fluorescent dye, indocyanine green (ICG). Chlorotoxin is a toxic small peptide (chain of amino acids) isolated from the venom of the Israeli death stalker scorpion, *Leiurus quinquestriatus*. The scorpion stores this venom in its telson (stinger) at the tip of its tail and uses it to immobilize and kill its prey.

On first read, it might seem scary to be using a scorpion toxin to light up human brain tumors. But tozuleristide is non-toxic. It is not the true scorpion venom. The chlorotoxin in tozuleristide is an inert, non-poisonous synthetic analog of the death stalker venom. It has been tested meticulously and found to be safe. Tozuleristide binds selectively to various primary brain tumors. When conjugated with the near infrared fluorescent dye ICG and administered intravenously to patients prior to surgery, it has been found to light up selected tumors bright green when they are visualized with a specialized fluorescent microscope. We were studying the efficacy of tozuleristide in aiding the visualization and resection of primary brain tumors in children. Carter and his family had volunteered for the study, and he had been randomized to the cohort in the study to receive the intravenous drug on the morning of surgery.

Once all the pre-op details had been worked out, the anesthesia team took Carter back to room 408 in the OR. Richard wept as he waved goodbye to his younger son. He told me later that he felt weightless at the time, as if he was on a roller coaster. He had no control over what was happening. He felt as if the floor beneath him had disappeared and he was falling. Things felt surreal to him.

Tobi put on a gown and accompanied Carter into the surgical suite. She watched as the team transferred him onto the OR table. Through tears, Carter told his mother that he loved her. She kissed his forehead while the anesthesiologist placed a mask over his face. He was asleep in a matter of seconds. A nurse escorted Tobi out of the OR and back to the waiting room. As soon as she saw Richard, she began sobbing loudly and uncontrollably. She and Richard took some belongings to the car and then sat down in the cafeteria for a bit but were too upset to eat. They went for a walk, prayed, paced, and waited anxiously for the operation to end, trying as best they could to distract themselves.

In the OR, we positioned Carter supine, with his head turned so that the right side was up, and we proceeded with the eviction of Carl from the right frontal lobe of Carter's brain. After localizing the tumor with our computer-based image guidance system, we made a lazy-S incision in the scalp behind Carter's hairline, just above and in front of his right ear. I performed the operation with our pediatric neurosurgery fellow, Andrew Kobets. Andrew was a superb neurosurgeon who did his residency training at the Albert Einstein College of Medicine with his mentor, Jim Goodrich, a world-class pediatric neurosurgeon and a close friend of mine. At the completion of his year-long fellowship with us at Johns Hopkins, Andrew was planning to return to Einstein to join the faculty and work with Jim as his mentor. Sadly, within the year, Jim became an early victim of the ravages of the COVID-19 pandemic and died of respiratory failure. It was a devastating loss for his family, friends, colleagues, students, and patients. Andrew would return to Einstein as Jim's replacement, rather than his understudy.

We performed a right frontal craniotomy, removing a trapdoor segment of the skull, and then localized the tumor using ultrasonography and frameless stereotactic image guidance. Working under microsurgical magnification, we opened the dura mater, the tough fibrous covering of the brain, to expose the cerebral cortex, the surface of the right frontal lobe of the brain. We made a small opening in the cerebral cortex and came down to the lesion. It was a dark burgundy mass that had the appearance of a large mulberry. It looked like a tangle of multiple blood vessels. The brain surrounding the mass was discolored and appeared greenish yellow, as if there had been a previous hemorrhage. This was a surprise. It didn't look anything like the low-grade glioma we were expecting. Instead, it looked like a cavernous vascular malformation surrounded by breakdown products of old blood.

Next, the PNOC team took intraoperative photographs of the lesion through the specialized microscopic filter and found that it fluoresced avidly, turning bright green and lighting up like a Christmas tree. There was no fluorescence of the surrounding brain tissue.

We were stymied. This was the fluorescence we were expecting if the mass was a low-grade brain tumor. But we could see with our eyes that there was no brain tumor. This was a vascular malformation. We accidentally stumbled on a novel finding, that tozuleristide not only lights up brain tumors, but vascular malformations as well. It was the first demonstration of fluorescence of a vascular malformation with tozuleristide and may suggest a wider role for this agent in surgery for different conditions.

We completed the surgery and removed the vascular malformation, using intraoperative electrophysiological monitoring of the motor cortex to help protect it from injury during the resection. At the end of the operation, we placed a white turban dressing on Carter's head and gave it a little flair by decorating it with "bear ears." He was extubated in the OR and transferred to the PICU at 3:30 p.m., where his parents visited with him.

Carter was groggy as he emerged from anesthesia but was awake enough to tell his family he loved them. We breathed a deep sigh of relief when we heard him speak. Initially, he had a little trouble getting his words out, but his language function normalized later in the day. He was able to move all his limbs off the bed, though he did have some weakness of the left side of his face, presumably due to the proximity of the mass to the right motor cortex. The facial weakness subsequently resolved three days later.

Carter drifted off to sleep as I explained to his parents that Carl was not a tumor but actually a cerebrovascular malformation. The finding was unexpected, but the lesion had been removed. Carter woke up several hours later. He called out for his dad, who was standing beside him, while Tobi was standing at the foot of the bed. "I'm really scared," he told them. "I don't know what to do." His parents asked him what he was scared about.

"I'm afraid about the operation," he told them. Tobi and Richard smiled and told Carter that the operation was over. He was surprised and relieved. He didn't even realize he'd had the surgery. He asked for his older brother, Lucas, who would come to visit him the following day dressed as a dinosaur. Carter was a very sweet young man. He thanked us for saving his life. Within minutes, he fell back asleep.

The next day, post-op day one, Carter was more alert and interactive. He was transferred out of the ICU to a regular room on the floor. He had a headache that he rated seven on a scale of ten, but that subsequently went down to zero after Tylenol. A repeat MRI confirmed that the lesion had been totally removed. Tobi and Richard brought Lucas to visit him. Lucas was impressed with Carter's bear ears head turban. Carter wanted to go for a walk in the hallway with Lucas but thought that they should both look alike. There was no gauze in the room for Lucas to fashion a headwrap of his own, so instead he took Carter's white plastic urinal seat, turned it upside down on his head, and donned a hospital gown to go for a stroll with his brother. The brothers had a strong bond. Fortunately, the plastic urinal had not yet been used.

Carter had a smooth post-op course. He had a poor appetite on the first two days after surgery, but by postop day three, he was hungry as a bear and downed a bacon cheeseburger. Pathology returned cavernous vascular malformation, confirming what we saw in the OR during the resection. He was discharged home on post-op day five.

Tobi noted that on the trip home, Carter was five different kids in five minutes in the car. He beamed when he got into the parking lot, and his smile broadened when he got in the car, and his mood elevated rapidly along the ride. As soon as they arrived home at their townhouse, Carter was glowing and dashed up the stairs. He was overjoyed to be home. It was familiar territory. He was grateful to have made it out of the hospital. Kids often improve dramatically, more than one might expect, once they return to a familiar environment. The psychology of safety is a powerful force in the process of healing.

Once he got over the excitement of being home, Carter became frustrated. He wanted to return immediately to the life he had before surgery. But he got tired quickly. And his hands were clumsy.

He tried to assemble a Lego pizza truck he had won in a bingo game at the hospital but had trouble even picking up the pieces, and he fumbled just trying to snap them together. Lucas sat patiently with him and helped him finish the puzzle. But his manual dexterity improved rapidly, and by two weeks after surgery, Carter's fine motor control was back. A friend of the family had given him a Nanoblock Titanic Lego set with over two thousand small pieces. He was able to complete it deftly in a couple of days, after finishing his schoolwork.

I saw Carter in follow-up six weeks later, and he was doing fine. He showed me some photos of his Halloween costume that year. He decided to dress up as a member of the Delta Force, carrying a plastic rifle squirt gun, wearing combat fatigues, and covering his face with green and black camouflage paint. But the high point of his outfit was what he had done with the nicely healing incision we had meticulously crafted for him on the right side of his scalp. He had carefully covered it with dripping red dye to make it look like a real battle wound. I complimented him on his creativity but asked him not to tell anyone that I was his surgeon because of concern that his friends and family would consider me to be a butcher based on his costume. The Paxtons brought me an unforgettable gift, a book entitled *The King and I*, with a picture of me they inserted next to Elvis on the title page. They were an incredibly kind family and brought homemade cupcakes for the doctors and nurses at Johns Hopkins who cared for Carter, and for Dr. Solowski as well.

In neurosurgery, we are often called on to make a clinical diagnosis based on the best information available at the time, usually the patient's history, physical exam, and imaging studies. Although we strive for accuracy, medicine is often fraught with uncertainty. This was the case with Carter Paxton. Based on the best available information, the number-one diagnosis for his incidental finding on the MRI was a brain tumor, likely a low-grade glioma. But at surgery, it turned out that diagnosis was incorrect—the lesion was a vascular malformation that mimicked a tumor. It's important to remember that we make a clinical diagnosis on the basis of probability. There's always a differential diagnosis, a list of other possibilities, including things such as inflammation, infection, and vascular anomalies. Based on probability, a tumor was the most likely diagnosis.

Carter was lucky. Although the actual diagnosis was cavernous vascular malformation, the treatment would have been the same if it were a tumor. The vascular malformation was accessible and needed to come out. It had bled previously and could have bled again. The surgical excision will prevent it from rebleeding.

In the process of removing Carter's cavernous vascular malformation, we made a serendipitous finding. We discovered by accident that tozuleristide (so-called "Tumor Paint") actually binds to cerebral vascular malformations in a similar way that it binds to brain tumors. We published this finding in the journal *Neurosurgery*. For Carter's case, the dye helped us define the margins of the resection, though Carter's surgery was relatively straightforward. But the binding of tozuleristide to vascular lesions may have future implications for fluorescence-guided surgery for patients with larger malformations with more complex geometry.

The finding is something we stumbled on unexpectedly. It was a fluke. It was the result of serendipity, a happy accident, an unplanned, fortunate discovery. Our small finding was of great interest to us, but its significance in the field of fluorescence-guided surgery has yet to be determined. Nevertheless, the contribution of serendipity in discovery should not be dismissed.

Over time, serendipity has played a powerful role in science and medicine. Its history is fascinating. The word was coined on January 28, 1754, by the English writer Horace Walpole, the youngest son of the British Prime Minister Robert Walpole, in a letter to his friend and distant relative Horace Mann, a British diplomat. He recounted a Persian folktale, *The Three Princes of Serendip* (modern-day Sri Lanka), who traveled the world making unusual discoveries by accident.

While our small finding in Carter's case may or may not prove to have some value over time, there are several legendary cases of serendipity in medicine. Perhaps the most famous is the discovery of the drug penicillin in September 1928 by the Scottish physician and bacteriologist, Alexander Fleming. He was working in his laboratory at St. Mary's Hospital in Paddington, London, at the time. He had been studying the influenza virus and had accidentally left a petri dish growing the bacterium, *Staphylococcus aureus*, uncovered on a lab bench near an open window instead of placing it in an incubator.

When he returned from a two-week vacation at his home in Scotland, he noted that there was an area on the petri dish where the staphylococci were not growing. That area had been contaminated by a blue-green fungus, which was surrounded by a bacteria-free circle. He suspected that the fungus contained an agent that killed the bacteria. Fleming identified the fungus as *Penicillium notatum* and isolated the "mold juice" from it, realizing that it had antibacterial effects. He named the extract penicillin and published his findings the following year in the *British Journal of Experimental Pathology*, though early on, it received little attention.

It wasn't until years later, during World War II, that penicillin achieved widespread use as an antibiotic, when techniques were developed to allow it to be mass-produced. By the end of the war, pharmaceutical companies were producing penicillin at the rate of 650 billion units a month. Fleming shared the Nobel Prize for his work with two others in 1945. It is estimated that since its discovery, the wonder drug penicillin has been responsible for saving over two hundred million lives. Fleming's observation was a landmark discovery—the identification of the world's first antibiotic—that changed the course of medicine. And it happened by chance. Fleming modestly said, "One sometimes finds what one is not looking for. Nature makes penicillin. I just found it."

Another example of serendipity in medicine is the finding of an association between the bacterium *Heliobacter pylori (H. pylori)* and gastritis and peptic ulcer disease. Credit for that finding goes to Robin Warren and Barry Marshall. At the time, Warren was a clinical pathologist in Perth, Australia. On the afternoon of June 11, 1979, his forty-second birthday, he was looking at a routine gastric biopsy under the microscope in his pathology laboratory when he saw something unusual.

What he saw was chronic gastritis (inflammation of the lining of the stomach) but also numerous small, curved bacilli (rod-shaped bacteria) growing on the surface of the stomach biopsy. That was an odd finding, he thought, because the conventional wisdom was that the stomach's acid environment made it sterile, such that no bacteria could survive there. Warren's finding reminds me of the words of Louis Pasteur at a lecture he gave in 1854 at the University of Lille, France, where he was professor of chemistry and dean of the science faculty: "In the field of observation, chance favors the prepared mind."

Warren was intrigued and reviewed prior gastric biopsies and found the spiral bacteria in multiple specimens. These organisms were difficult to see using the conventional hematoxylin and eosin (H&E) stains, but Warren was a passionate photographer and developed a novel silver stain that lit up the specimens vividly. Warren was intrigued by his finding, but unfortunately, other investigators were unable to confirm it. He faced disbelief and even hostility. A close colleague described his work to him: "It's just rubbish." The same colleague noted that Warren would often take his work home, sitting at his microscope "till two in the morning, then come to work the next day and fall asleep."

Warren was confident in his observations but realized they were counter to the standard teaching that nothing can grow in the stomach. The prevailing opinion was that peptic ulcer disease was caused by an acid environment made worse by stress or psychiatric disease. At one point, he felt his wife, Winifred, an accomplished psychiatrist, was the only person who believed him. "She stood beside me and helped me when no one else would," he said.

A few years later, in 1981, a young gastroenterology fellow named Barry Marshall was looking for a research project and was guided to Warren by his department chair to see if there was any substance to "that mad pathologist's claims." Marshall was not very enthusiastic about the project, but over time became intrigued and worked with Warren to collect more clinical data. The bacterial organism was elusive, and they had difficulty growing it on agar plates. Fortuitously, the plates were left unattended in an incubator for several days over the Easter holiday in 1982, allowing enough time for the small bacterial colonies to flourish. The organism was ultimately named *Heliobacter pylori*.

In a remarkable episode of self-experimentation, Marshall, who had been frustrated by the lack of an animal model for the disease, decided to infect himself with *H. pylori*. First, he underwent an endoscopic biopsy on himself to prove that the lining of his stomach was normal. He then drank a beaker filled with *H. pylori* obtained from an infected patient. Eight days later, he became haggard and cranky, with uncontrollable vomiting every morning. He described his breath as "like a sewer," a finding that bothered his wife even more than it bothered him. He underwent repeat gastroscopy on himself, which now demonstrated gastritis and the offending *H. pylori* microbe, after which he took antibiotics and recovered. In 2005, Warren and Marshall were awarded the Nobel Prize for Physiology or Medicine for their pioneering work allowing the disabling condition of peptic ulcer disease to be treated with a regimen of antibiotics and acid secretion inhibitors.

Yet another example of serendipity in medicine is the discovery of the role of sildenafil citrate (brand name Viagra) as a treatment for erectile dysfunction (ED). Epidemiologic data suggest that ED is a widespread problem affecting many men, with a prevalence of up to 33 percent in the United States. An early and particularly dramatic example of the use of medication to treat ED was demonstrated by the clever but eccentric British neurophysiologist Professor Giles Brindley on April 18, 1983. He was giving an hour-long invited lecture about ED at 7 p.m. at the annual meeting of the American Urological Society in Las Vegas, Nevada. There were several hundred people in the audience for the session, including surgeons, researchers, and spouses. The audience included the twelve other speakers to follow him, though no one in the audience would remember anything the other speakers had to say.

Members of the audience were dressed in formal evening attire and thought it was a bit odd when Brindley took the stage in casual gym clothes and began by showing a series of slides of penile erections in various stages following pharmacological injections. The mixed audience was in a state of shock when he announced that the pictures were of himself.

To further prove his point, Brindley had injected himself directly into his own penis with the drug phenoxybenzamine, an alpha-adrenergic blocker used to treat some forms of hypertension. He then stood to the side of the podium, demonstrating to his astonished audience the bulge in his sweatpants. In case anyone had any doubts, he then dropped his pants and his undershorts to exhibit his erect penis in the flesh.

He then left the stage and walked in the aisles among the audience to a combination of gasps, screams, and laughter. Some thought he was an exhibitionist. Many thought he was an oddball British scientist. But his contribution introduced a new era in the treatment of ED. Years later, he was knighted by the queen. To say that Brindley gave a memorable talk is an understatement. One can't help but feel sorry for the poor speaker who had to talk after him. It certainly put a new meaning to the phrase, "This is a hard act to follow."

Brindley believed that the mechanism of action was that the drug caused relaxation of the smooth muscle in the blood vessels of the corpus cavernosum, the spongy erectile tissue in the shaft of the penis. Subsequently, researchers began focusing on the physiology of the penile erection, searching for the factor responsible for penile smooth muscle cell dilation. That factor turned out to be nitric oxide, and emphasizing the importance of that discovery, in 1992, the journal *Science* identified nitric oxide as its "Molecule of the Year."

Sildenafil citrate is a potent vasodilator that works by stimulating the release of nitric oxide. It was being investigated as a means of treating angina pectoris, chest pain due to inadequate blood flow to the heart. In the late 1980s, the pharmaceutical company Pfizer was investigating the vasodilating effects of sildenafil in the treatment of patients with angina. The drug had only minimal effects on the heart, but nurses noted that several of the male patients were lying prone during the study. The reason was that many of them were embarrassed to have developed erections from the penile vasodilatory effects of sildenafil.

This chance serendipitous observation of the effects of sildenafil on the penis rather than the heart led to the development of an entirely new industry that revolutionized the treatment of ED with the oral agent Viagra and similar-acting pharmaceuticals. In its second year on the market, Viagra brought in over $1 billion in global sales. In 1998, the scientists Robert Furchgott, Louis Ignarro, and Ferid Murad shared the Nobel Prize for their elucidation of the mechanism of nitric oxide, the chemical that led to Viagra.

Some may feel that because serendipitous findings occur by accident, they should not be considered a form of true science. I believe the exact opposite is true. Most breakthroughs in science and medicine don't occur as the result of a eureka moment. They are often the result of painstaking methodical investigation, in which experiments intended to confirm predicted outcomes occasionally fail. The ability to recognize the potential significance of unexpected findings can sometimes lead to extraordinary discovery. In the words of Albert Szent-Gyorgi, the Hungarian biochemist who won the Nobel Prize in 1937 for discoveries elucidating the function of vitamin C, "Discovery consists of seeing what everybody has seen and thinking what nobody has thought."

Carter is now nineteen years old and has graduated from high school. He is taking a gap year before going off to college and is learning how to drive. He hopes to major in marine biology because he has always had a love of the ocean and is considering a career helping injured sea animals recover. He is also thinking about the possibility of becoming a psychotherapist. It was a traumatic and terrifying experience for Carter to undergo brain surgery as a twelve-year-old boy. Even after he was discharged from the hospital, he would often tear up when friends and family asked him about his experience. He saw a therapist for several weeks, who helped him get back on track with meditation, visual imagery, and music. He feels that becoming a therapist would afford him the opportunity to give back to others facing similar stresses.

Today, Carter is a perfectly normal young man except that he can't smell a thing. He still has a bowl of cereal for breakfast each morning but decided to switch from Cinnamon Toast Crunch to Cheerios in an effort to follow a healthier diet. Whenever the milk tastes even the slightest bit funny, he calls over a family member to make sure it hasn't gone sour. His mom documented his experience in a Facebook blog called *Grateful for Spoiled Milk*.

"I am thankful that my family was with me all the way," Carter said. "Once in a while, I touch my scar and think about all that has happened in my life. I'm aware that Carl (the name he gave to his tumor/vascular malformation) could have done me in. I'm grateful to have a second chance at life.

And I believe that this all happened because God wanted to save my life by spoiling some milk."

CHAPTER 16

Tip of the Iceberg

"How the seen looks depends on how the seer sees."

Mokokoma Mokhonoana
Philosopher and Social Critic
Limpopo, South Africa
November 2020

It was early in the morning on Thursday, October 29, 2020, and my day was getting off to a slow start in the hospital. Things took a sudden turn when I was summoned urgently to the Johns Hopkins Emergency Room to consult on a child who was unresponsive with a large brain tumor. That's how I first met young Daniel Adekanmbi, who at the time was lying on his back on a stretcher, stuporous with his eyes closed, barely responsive. I got the story from the ER team and from Daniel's mother, Olubisi, who sat beside him, exhausted, having been awake the entire night.

Daniel was a seven-year-old right-handed boy who had been in excellent health previously. He was a happy child and a good student in the third grade. The COVID-19 pandemic was in full force, so all schooling was being done online from home. Olubisi first noticed that there was something wrong with Daniel two weeks earlier when he awakened in the morning feeling punky with a low-grade fever. She brought him to an urgent care facility, where he was diagnosed with a viral illness. He was tested for COVID-19 and found to be negative. A respiratory viral panel was normal, as were routine blood tests.

Olubisi brought Daniel home, where he wasn't able to do much of anything. He continued to feel lousy and complained of a headache and nausea with chills and sweats. His fever continued, and he had several bouts of vomiting, which continued each day. He couldn't eat much, and he felt very weak. He was too sick to go online for school. All he could do was lie around and rest.

The headache persisted and worsened each day. One week before Daniel's admission to Johns Hopkins, Olubisi brought him to a local hospital. He complained of headache, vomiting, and fatigue. He still had fever, though his temperature would come down temporarily with Tylenol. Blood tests sent from the ER were normal. The ER team thought he was constipated and released him. Olubisi didn't agree with the diagnosis but didn't know what was wrong. She brought Daniel home, where he remained bedridden with the same complaints, unable to do much of anything.

Then, in the early hours of Thursday morning, October 29, just after midnight, Daniel awakened to go to the bathroom. He had been vomiting and felt light-headed when he got up. He summoned Olubisi, who helped him walk to the bathroom.

When Daniel began to pee, he became more lightheaded and collapsed to the floor, where he was unresponsive and apneic (not breathing). Olubisi couldn't feel a pulse. She initiated cardiopulmonary resuscitation (CPR) immediately, including chest compression and mouth-to-mouth breathing, while simultaneously asking one of her other sons to call 911. She had learned the technique as a nursing student. She was scared out of her mind. Moments ago, she was fast asleep, and here she was performing CPR on her little boy. It was surreal. She thought he was going to die.

She continued the CPR for what felt like an eternity but was actually about five minutes. She stopped when she saw Daniel start to breathe on his own. The emergency medical technicians came quickly, gave Daniel intravenous fluids and oxygen, and brought him to the ER of another local hospital. Olubisi accompanied them in the ambulance and asked her neighbor to keep an eye on her other kids. Everything had happened incredibly quickly. Olubisi was in a state of panic, shaking with fear.

The doctors in the ER resuscitated Daniel further with a liter of intravenous glucose and saline, along with ondansetron, an antiemetic agent. They sent him for an emergency head CT scan. The CT showed a large tumor at the base of Daniel's brain along with hydrocephalus, an accumulation of cerebrospinal fluid in the cerebral ventricles. They gave him an intravenous dose of dexamethasone, a steroid, before sending him off to us at Johns Hopkins for further management.

I was summoned to see Daniel in the Hopkins ER that morning when he arrived. I got more history from Olubisi. Daniel lived with her and his three brothers—Walter, William, and his twin David on Quilting Bee Road in Catonsville, Maryland. Daniel and David were dizygotic (fraternal) twins, meaning there were two separate eggs fertilized by two separate sperm cells. Daniel was born in Lagos, Nigeria. The pregnancy was uncomplicated. He was delivered at term via cesarean section as twin B with a birth weight of 2.3 kilograms. His brother David was twin A and weighed 2.7 kilograms.

Two years earlier, when Daniel was five, Olubisi obtained a visa, packed up her four young boys, and moved to the United States in hopes of creating a better life for them. She chose to come to Maryland because she had read about it and thought it sounded like a good state. Her husband, Adelaja, was unable to get a visa and remained in Lagos, where he continues to work as an engineer. He is hoping to come to the US soon. In the meantime, he communicates with his family digitally on WhatsApp.

It was a tough struggle for Olubisi when she arrived in the US alone with her kids and no resources. She found employment working nights as a caregiver in a group home. At the same time, she spent two years attending nursing school and got her degree. Currently, she works at the Autumn Lake Nursing Home in Catonsville.

Daniel's developmental milestones had been normal. The only health problem Olubisi remembered him having was an episode of headache, vomiting, and fever that occurred two years earlier when they lived in Nigeria, just before moving to the US. Daniel was hospitalized and diagnosed with malaria. He was treated with hydroxychloroquine and antibiotics and got better over a period of about two weeks.

I examined Daniel in the ER. He remained deeply unresponsive but occasionally opened his eyes and withdrew his arms and legs to painful stimuli. He didn't talk or interact with me. I reviewed the CT with my neurosurgical colleagues. There was an unusual-appearing, large, roundish, multilobulated mass in Daniel's cerebellum at the base of his brain. It was compressing the fourth ventricle, causing hydrocephalus, with enlargement of the lateral and third ventricles and resultant increased intracranial pressure. The increased pressure contributed to Daniel's altered mental status. So did the fact that he had just sustained a cardiopulmonary arrest from which he was resuscitated by his mother.

But something else on the CT caught our eye. With careful inspection, we also identified a small, subtle fullness in the midline of the soft tissues of the scalp, just outside the skull, adjacent to the underlying tumor. I went back to examine Daniel further. Looking at the back of his head, I noticed a tiny midline dimple. It was dark, barely visible, only about a millimeter in diameter. I asked Olubisi if this area had ever swelled up in the past and if there had ever been any drainage from the dimple.

"Yes, that little spot has been there since Daniel was born. It swells up from time to time. It comes and goes. But I haven't seen any drainage." She said she hadn't given it much thought in the past.

That tiny midline dimple would prove to be the key finding in diagnosing the mass in Daniel's brain. It was the tip of the iceberg. We suspected that the dimple was a portal of entry to a dermal sinus, a narrow abnormal conduit that connected the scalp to the brain. A dermal sinus is a skin-like tract that dives deep in the midline through the soft tissue, penetrating the skull, ending up in the brain as a large cyst filled with sebaceous material (oily fat) and keratin, a natural protein.

We ordered an emergency MRI to better define the mass in Daniel's brain. Because he had lost consciousness, we intubated him and administered general anesthesia to control his ventilation for the MRI.

Cranial dermoid cysts have a characteristic appearance on MRI. They occur in the midline and are well-circumscribed. On diffusion weighted imaging (DWI) sequences of the MRI, they show restriction of diffusion. DWI measures the dispersion of water by analyzing the small, random Brownian movements of water molecules. Restriction of diffusion is often seen in malignant tumors because of their high cellularity. Although dermoid cysts are benign, they too can restrict diffusion because of their thickened cyst contents.

The MRI confirmed our suspicion. It showed a sinus tract extending from the tiny midline dimple in the skin, passing deep through the skull, ending in a large cyst in the midline of the base of the brain. The cyst had likely ruptured to cause an inflammatory reaction in the surrounding brain. The mass had blocked the outflow for the fourth ventricle, causing severe obstructive hydrocephalus, much like a ball can block the drain of a sink, causing water from the faucet to overflow. Because of the increased pressure in Daniel's head, the cerebellum had herniated downward, through the foramen magnum, the opening at the base of the skull, and was compressing the brainstem and spinal cord, likely contributing further to his poor mental status.

The tipoff to the diagnosis was the finding of the small midline scalp dimple in the setting of fever, headache, vomiting, and a midline mass in the cerebellum on CT and MRI. Brain tumors don't usually cause fever. But a midline dimple can be the opening of a sinus tract in the skin that results from incomplete separation of the neural tube in embryologic development. In other words, there is persistence of an embryonic connection between the skin and the brain.

This was a congenital malformation, an abnormality Daniel had been born with. The sinus tract dived deeply, penetrated the skull and terminated in a large cyst in the brain. The sinus tract can act as a portal of entry for bacteria from the skin to the brain. Daniel's fever could have been caused by organisms from the skin entering the cyst through the sinus tract, causing meningitis or a brain abscess. The fever could also have been secondary to rupture of the cyst, causing chemical inflammation of the surrounding brain from release of the irritative cyst contents.

As soon as the MRI was completed, we took Daniel directly to the OR. Olubisi gave him a kiss and said a tearful goodbye, still overcome by fear. Assisting me in the case were two superb neurosurgeons, Kurt Lehner and Jignesh Tailor.

First, with Daniel asleep and supine, we made a small opening in the right side of his skull and placed a catheter into his enlarged lateral ventricle to drain the cerebrospinal fluid. The pressure was sky high, and we brought it down with drainage. Next, with Daniel in the prone position, we went after the dermal sinus and dermoid cyst. I remember looking at the diminutive midline dimple on the back of Daniel's head after his hair was shaved. It was hard to believe that this tiny pinpoint punctum, which could easily have been overlooked, could be the source of so much mischief. It emphasizes the importance of a careful physical exam, even in the age of technology, with all the impressive diagnostic tools available to us.

We opened the back of Daniel's head, taking care to make a small ellipse in the skin and trace the dermal sinus down through the skull all the way into the brain, carefully making a craniotomy to facilitate the exposure. We also removed a small posterior portion of the atlas (the first cervical bone) because the mass had squeezed the brain downward through the foramen magnum, the large opening in the base of the skull, where it caused pressure on the brainstem and spinal cord. The dermoid cyst in the brain was surrounded by an arachnoid cyst, another congenital fluid collection. The brain looked angry. It appeared that the dermoid cyst had ruptured at some point and was densely adherent to the surrounding cerebellum, causing significant inflammation.

We opened up the dermoid cyst capsule to decompress it and encountered thick, viscous, yellowish material with sebaceous gland secretions, oil, fat, and small strands of hair. The operation was difficult, but we were able to dissect the dermoid cyst off the cerebellum and remove the cyst and sinus tract completely.

I went to speak to Olubisi in the waiting room. It was late in the evening. We had been in the OR for almost nine hours. Olubisi had spent the time pacing, crying, and praying. She was alone and fearful. She was too anxious to eat anything. She didn't know if Daniel was going to survive the surgery.

I explained to Olubisi that we found the dermal sinus and dermoid cyst and that we were able to remove it all. The pressure was off the brain, but there was a lot of inflammation and scar tissue due to prior rupture of the cyst. We would need to treat Daniel with antibiotics to prevent infection and steroids to prevent inflammation. With guarded optimism, I told Olubisi I thought Daniel was going to be okay, but that we would likely go through a stormy few weeks during the recovery.

I brought Olubisi to see Daniel in the PICU. The breathing tube was still in place, but he had his eyes open and was slowly awakening from anesthesia, moving his limbs. He recognized his mom. Olubisi cried and gave him a kiss. She was relieved to see him alive and responsive. Because it was late at night and the operation had been long and difficult, we decided to keep Daniel sedated. We left the breathing tube in place overnight for fear that his respiratory effort might not be strong enough if we extubated him too early. We also left his ventricular drain open to keep the intracranial pressure controlled.

Daniel made a smooth recovery, and we were able to extubate him after twenty-four hours. He began eating and playing on his iPad. He had some dysmetria (incoordination) in his right arm, likely from irritation of his cerebellum. The dysmetria cleared over about ten days. We were able to wean Daniel from the externalized ventricular drain and removed it after several days. Pathology returned dermal sinus and dermoid cyst with inflammation, as we had expected. He got a little better each day and was walking independently when we discharged him home two weeks after his surgery.

But Daniel had a bit of a stormy course. He returned three days after discharge with fever and swelling underneath the incision in the back of his head. He had developed a pseudomeningocele underneath his incision, an accumulation of cerebrospinal fluid that leaked through a small pinhole opening that developed at the site of our dural closure. The inflamed cerebellum caused a blockage in his cerebrospinal fluid pathways even after the mass had been removed, and his hydrocephalus returned. We had to go back and repair the leak in his dura and ultimately place a ventriculoperitoneal shunt to treat the hydrocephalus and keep the pressure off his brain.

It was a difficult few weeks for Daniel, who had to undergo two subsequent procedures after our initial resection of his dermal sinus and dermoid cyst. And things weren't easy for Olubisi, who had to bring Daniel back and forth to the hospital while caring for her three other sons and continuing to work at her job in a local nursing home. The fact that this was all going on in the middle of the COVID-19 pandemic didn't make things any easier.

Somehow, after a long slog, everything worked out. Daniel recovered. He was back to his old self. He had no headache, no vomiting, and no fever. His mental fogginess resolved. He was off all medication. And his MRI was clean, with no evidence of any residual or recurrent mass and no hydrocephalus.

I have continued to follow Daniel in our outpatient clinic and was pleased to see him return to normal. But two years after his original surgery, he began complaining of headaches again. These were not as severe as they had been at the time of his initial presentation to us, but they persisted and came on daily. This time, he had no fever. Initially, we were concerned that there might be a fragment of his dermoid cyst that had not been removed and had grown. But serial post-op MRIs had been normal, with no sign of residual or recurrent dermoid.

Olubisi noticed that the headaches seemed to be worse when Daniel was upright and active and improved when he laid down. We repeated an MRI, which confirmed that the dermoid was gone. But his cerebral ventricles had become small and slit-like. Our suspicion was that his ventricular shunt, which transported the fluid from his ventricles to be absorbed by blood vessels in his peritoneum, was overdraining.

Fortunately, that was an easy problem to fix. When we had inserted the ventriculoperitoneal shunt, we placed a programmable valve in the system. By placing a magnet on top of Daniel's head directly over the shunt valve, we could change the valve setting, adding more resistance into the system without having to go back to the OR. That worked. His headaches resolved, and a repeat MRI showed that his ventricles were no longer slit-like and had increased to an appropriate size.

Daniel's congenital occipital dermal sinus/dermoid cyst is an exceedingly rare entity. These benign lesions can occur anywhere along the neuraxis (central nervous system), usually in the midline, and account for less than 0.5 percent of all brain tumors. Dermoid cysts are atypical neoplasms. They don't enlarge the way most tumors grow, by cells continuing to divide. Rather, they enlarge in a linear fashion by desquamation (shedding of dead epithelial cells from the cyst lining) and secretion of glandular substances.

The majority of dermal sinus tracts and cysts occur in the spine. Those that are cranial in location are usually in the back of the head, as was the case with Daniel's lesion. Very rarely, they can occur as a tiny punctum at the tip of the nose, tracking subcutaneously up through the base of the skull into the brain, ending in a cyst.

Dermal sinuses are often clinically occult, as was the case with Daniel, whose tiny midline occipital dimple could have easily been overlooked. Sometimes, these lesions are discovered after a child has unexplained recurrent bouts of bacterial meningitis or brain abscess. Occasionally, they come to attention because of recurrent headaches and fevers from cyst rupture, creating aseptic (chemical) meningitis from inflammation caused by the spilled cyst contents. Though rare, these dermal sinus lesions should be considered in the differential diagnosis of a midline cerebellar mass in a child with headache and fever. The reason for this is that the management of these lesions is different from that of a conventional brain tumor.

The fact that we stumbled on a key finding in Daniel's case, the tiny midline pit on the back of his scalp, reminds me of the importance of bedside diagnosis. In the current age of technology, it is easy to see how one might jump from the patient's complaint directly to neuroimaging studies. But the physical exam remains essential. There is still an important human element in the detection of disorders of the nervous system.

I've had a longstanding interest in the history of neurosurgery. On my office wall, there are old photographs of three neurosurgical giants: Harvey Cushing (the founder of modern neurosurgery), Franc Ingraham (the founder of pediatric neurosurgery and Cushing's disciple), and Donald Matson (master pediatric neurosurgeon and Ingraham's disciple). I didn't realize it until I looked up at them while writing this story that each of these pioneers is standing at the bedside examining a child with a neurologic disease. The photos convey a powerful message. Despite the enormous technological advances that have occurred in medicine, we should not forget the art of bedside diagnosis and localization. There is still much to be gleaned from a careful history and physical exam.

I remember a conversation I had with Robin Humphreys over a decade ago. He was a mentor, friend, and distinguished professor of neurosurgery at the Hospital for Sick Children in Toronto. He had just given a major presentation about neurosurgical innovation at the annual meeting of the American Association of Neurological Surgeons. I had asked him a question, and he was waxing philosophical about the benefits and detriments of the modernization of our field. He quoted the insightful counsel of a former chair of pediatrics from Canada: "Don't just do something! Stand there and observe the child."

The power of observation should not be forgotten. My patient Daniel had been sent to us from an outside hospital for management of a posterior fossa brain tumor. The subtle extracranial findings on his original outside head CT had not been noted. It's understandable why. The large intracranial mass was the elephant in the room, and in the chaotic environment of the referring hospital ER, the goal was to stabilize Daniel and transfer him to us as quickly and safely as possible—which is exactly what they did.

Our discovery of Daniel's midline scalp dimple was fortuitous and emphasizes the importance of the human touch in making a clinical diagnosis. The powerful CT scan must be interpreted in the context of the presenting illness. The doctor still plays a fundamental role in diagnosis and treatment. And a paramount role in the process of healing.

But with artificial intelligence (AI) barreling down the pike, the landscape may be changing. AI is rapidly changing the way we do things in my field. That's not to say that AI will ever replace the role of the physician. I don't think that will ever happen. But I believe AI will unquestionably change the way we practice medicine. And if harnessed thoughtfully, AI has the potential to make exponential improvements in the way we care for our neurosurgical patients. I believe it will play a major role in patient management before, during, and after surgery.

Consider, for example, the challenges in diagnosing the rare dermal sinus and dermoid cyst for our patient Daniel. AI, with its capacity to analyze and learn from extensive datasets, could have the ability to identify selected patterns on neuroimaging studies more accurately than humans. The subtle findings on Daniel's original CT were not readily apparent. But suppose we could enter Daniel's symptoms and CT images into a computer with access to thousands of digitized scans for reference. Comparisons would be made with lightning speed. Such a processor could provide substantial assistance in differential diagnosis and treatment planning. I see AI as a powerful tool to support rather than replace the neurosurgeon.

We learn from our patients and do a fair amount of teaching at our academic medical center. Robert Heinlein, the influential American science-fiction author, put it nicely: "When one teaches, two learn."

We found a teachable moment caring for Daniel. In carefully reviewing his original CT, we noted something unusual about the bone at the base of his skull. Usually, the skull has a single midline internal occipital keel, or crest. Daniel's CT had two bony crests, one on either side of an internal midline depression in the skull. We surmised that Daniel's congenital midline occipital dermoid had caused local pressure because it had been present since birth. This caused scalloping of the overlying portion of the skull, creating two internal crests rather than the usual single midline crest.

We believed this observation was a useful radiographic sign heralding the presence of a longstanding midline brain abnormality, such as a dermoid, that had been present since birth. We struggled for a time to come up with a novel name for our new radiologic finding. Ultimately, we came to realize that the two raised crests surrounding the midline internal skull depression bore a striking resemblance to a predatory alligator lurking in the water with its eyes just above the surface. We engaged the services of Larry Lynch, an exceptional nature photographer, and placed a photo he took of a menacing alligator adjacent to Daniel's dermoid CT. We published an article describing the findings in the journal *Child's Nervous System*. The title of the article was "Alligator Eyes: Beware the Occipital Dermoid."

Daniel has continued to thrive. Five years after his surgery, he is in middle school, thirteen years old, and in the seventh grade, making the honor roll. His favorite teacher is Mr. Feix, who teaches gym class. His favorite subject is math, and his least favorite is language sciences ("it's boring"). He enjoys battling with his friends online, playing video games, particularly Fortnite. He also enjoys Roblox and Call of Duty. His favorite sport is soccer, but he also likes to play baseball, basketball, and kickball with his friends. His best friends Judah, Jackson, Shazab, and Ammar live close by and often play hide and seek, tag, or watch Netflix shows like *Fuller House* and *iCarly*. His appetite has returned, and his favorite food is spaghetti.

I asked him what he wants to do when he grows up. "I want to be a brain surgeon and save people's lives," he said decisively. "If that doesn't work out, I'll be a soccer star. Maybe I can do both." For reasons unclear to me, he's not my only patient aiming for a career path in brain surgery and soccer. But it's always good in life to have a backup plan.

CHAPTER 17

Postponing Death

"That it will never come again is
what makes life so sweet."

Emily Dickinson
"That It Will Never Come Again"
Poem 1741
Complete Poems

As a young child growing up in Poughkeepsie, New York, in the 1950s, my memories are happy ones. We didn't have video games, cell phones, or iPads in those days, but the kids in my neighborhood would often get together after school and on weekends to hang out. Sometimes we'd play outdoors, and sometimes we'd sit and watch TV. My favorite show was *The Adventures of Superman*, starring George Reeves in the title role. I watched the show religiously and felt it was my destiny to "fight a never-ending battle for truth, justice and the American way." In fact, I asked my mother to make me my own Superman outfit, consisting of a black cape and a gray suit. She told me the ensemble needed to have a red cape and a blue suit, the way Superman looked in the real world, or at least in the comic books. But I had never seen the comics. I only saw Superman on our TV, which was in black and white. So, against my mother's advice, I ran around the neighborhood as Superman, dressed in a black cape and a gray suit.

My friends and I were young and carefree in our elementary school days, and we played a variety of outdoor games, including hide and seek, tag, cops and robbers, and cowboys and Indians. It didn't matter what the game was—somehow, I would always show up as Superman. Maybe a psychoanalyst could draw a connection between my Superman childhood and my current career choice, but I just remember having fun as a kid. My memories, though somewhat faded over the decades, were joyful. I had never really had any significant experience with sadness or grief.

One of the kids I played with was Stuart Krauss, who lived a few blocks away. He was closer to my brother Jason, who was a year younger than me, but we all spent a lot of time together. Stewie, as we called him, was a sweet, happy-go-lucky little guy. He was a thin, scrawny kid who was small for his age, but he was one of the gang, and he was always fun to be around.

One day, when we called Stewie to come over and play, his mother told us he couldn't because he was sick. After that call, as best I can remember, Stewie never came out to play with us again. We learned he had bone cancer and was being treated with chemotherapy. I didn't really know what bone cancer meant, but I knew it was something bad, because the few times we did see Stewie in school, he was ashen with no hair on his head. And he had lost a lot of weight. He was away a lot, probably sick from his illness and his treatment. And then we never saw him again. He died young from a relentlessly progressive illness. It was my first experience with death. I was deeply troubled by the experience and remember it to this day.

Later, I would learn that Stewie died from metastatic Ewing sarcoma, an aggressive form of bone cancer. The disease was first described in 1921 by James Ewing, who became the first professor of pathology at the Cornell University Medical College, where I did my training. Ewing sarcoma is a highly lethal malignancy, though with advances in molecular biology and improvements in chemotherapy today, the survival rate for patients has improved significantly. Some patients can even be cured.

I still think about Stewie's illness. He was ravaged by the effects of his bone cancer, but also by the toxicities of the chemotherapy utilized to treat the disease. As a child, I didn't fully grasp the nature of this horrible sickness that had taken away our young friend. As a surgeon, I sometimes reflect on Stewie's life and recognize that, at times, we are confronted with diseases that cannot be cured. In such cases, we often turn our attention to preserving life and forestalling death. These efforts can still be extremely gratifying, but it is essential that they be focused not only on length of life but also on quality of life. It is a delicate balance, and no two cases are the same.

Efforts to postpone death date back to the beginning of the practice of medicine. The way we practice neurosurgery today is markedly different from the methods used at the field's inception. One thing that has not changed over the years, however, is the emotional intensity experienced by anyone who has ever been affected by a life-threatening illness. This holds true not only for the patient but also for family members, friends, and medical and nursing staff who have provided care throughout the ordeal. Much of what we do in neurosurgery deals with illnesses that are potentially fatal.

A memorable example of forestalling death played out at the dawn of the discipline of modern neurosurgery. The following narrative concerns two of the field's founding giants, Harvey Williams Cushing and Wilder Graves Penfield.

Harvey Cushing is the undisputed father of modern neurosurgery. After training at Johns Hopkins with the legendary William Stewart Halsted, the father of modern surgery, Cushing began to focus on surgical disorders of the nervous system in 1901. He did this against the advice of his mentor Halsted, who tried to dissuade him because the neurosurgical outcomes were unacceptably poor during the prior decade. But Cushing persevered, and his pioneering work at the beginning of the twentieth century established modern neurosurgery as a separate discipline. He described this new specialty in a landmark address to the Cleveland Academy of Medicine in 1904, calling it *The Special Field*.

Wilder Penfield graduated from Princeton in 1913 and obtained a Rhodes Scholarship to study at Oxford. He earned his medical degree from Johns Hopkins and became a disciple of Cushing, with whom he worked at the Peter Bent Brigham Hospital in Boston. He also studied in Europe with such luminaries as the British neurophysiologist Charles Sherrington, the Spanish neuroscientist Pio del Rio Hortega, the German neurosurgeon Fedor Krause, and the German neurologist and neurosurgeon, Otfrid Foerster.

During World War I, Penfield worked in a military hospital in France, where, in 1916, he was injured and shattered his left leg in an explosion from a torpedo attack on his ship in which several others were killed. He was rescued and had a prolonged recovery, spending weeks recuperating at the home of William Osler, with whom he had previously trained. In 1934, with funding from the Rockefeller Foundation, Penfield would go on to create the prestigious Montreal Neurological Institute. Both Cushing and Penfield were brilliant neurosurgeons who had great respect for one another, one as the mentor and the other as the mentee.

In 1928, Penfield moved to Montreal, where he became the first neurosurgeon in the city's history, working at the Royal Victoria Hospital. On December 11 of that year, when he was only thirty-seven years old, Penfield was forced to make the unimaginable decision to operate on his own sister, Ruth Inglis.

Ruth was forty-three years old at the time, six years senior to her neurosurgeon brother. She had suffered from headaches and seizures since she was a child. Her parents were God-fearing Christian Scientists and generally believed in healing through prayer. Penfield remembered standing outside his sister's room in horror as a thirteen-year-old boy, seeing her lying unconscious following a generalized tonic-clonic seizure. She had several more seizures over the ensuing years but was ultimately able to lead a relatively ordinary life, at least for a time. She married Jack Inglis, her former high school teacher, with whom she had six healthy children. She was a happy wife and mother.

As an adult living in Los Angeles, Ruth developed more frequent seizures along with worsening headaches and vomiting over a period of two years. At the urging of her family, she made the trip by train with her mother from LA to Montreal to meet with her younger brother, who had just begun working at the Royal Victoria. Penfield examined his sister, looking deep into her eyes with an ophthalmoscope, and saw papilledema, increased pressure on the heads of the optic nerves. He described how he felt in his autobiography, *No Man Alone*:

> "There, standing close to this sister of mine, of whom I had so many precious boyhood memories, I brought my right eye close to hers, pupil to pupil with only the lens of the ophthalmoscope between them. Sure enough! There it was! The swelling of the head of the optic nerve—dreadful swelling, and there were little red hemorrhages, each bordered by a white margin, that extended menacingly over the surface of the surrounding retina."

The eyes are a window to the brain, and Penfield realized immediately that Ruth had "a very high degree of pressure within the skull. It had gone too far. She might well go blind within a day or two." Realizing the gravity of the situation, he described how he felt when he saw his sister's papilledema: "My knees grew suddenly weak and for a moment I thought I might fall. I put my hand on Ruth's shoulder to steady myself and waited until control returned to my knees, pretending to study her retina. Then we went out into the hall, laughing at old jokes as in the old days, and down the stairs to breakfast."

Penfield sent his sister for skull X-rays at the Royal Victoria. The films showed calcium granules deep in the right frontal lobe outlining a large brain tumor. This was way back in 1928, when there was no CT or MRI to provide a more detailed roadmap of what was going on. It was clear that Ruth needed urgent surgery, and Penfield wanted to send her to Cushing in Boston for treatment of her large brain tumor before she would end up going blind or dying from increased intracranial pressure. But Penfield's colleagues in Montreal felt there was no time and urged him to do the operation himself, even though in his nascent career he had never previously removed a tumor this large. Penfield wrote, "A wise physician will never 'doctor' himself or members of his family if he can help it. And yet there are times that he must act."

And act he did, reluctantly carrying out the surgery on his sister through a right frontal craniotomy while she was awake under local anesthesia. It is curious that the brain, the seat of all sensation, does not feel pain. Only the scalp and the dura mater (Latin for "tough mother"), the fibrous lining surrounding the brain, have pain receptors. In fact, Penfield went on to make major contributions to the field of epilepsy surgery, one of which was to carry out selected surgeries using local anesthesia with the patient awake to protect vital brain function.

Penfield's operation on his sister was difficult, and he struggled in the OR for hours. The tumor was large and within the confines of the right frontal lobe of her brain. As he was removing the inferior portion of the tumor, he came upon enormous veins arising from the bottom of the frontal lobe. While separating the tumor from these veins, he suddenly encountered a rush of blood coming up and filling the wound. Ruth's pulse became thready, and her condition turned critical.

Penfield was alarmed. All of this was going on while his sister was awake but drifting off. She received an emergency blood transfusion and began to stabilize. Penfield was finally able to stop the bleeding by applying pressure with a large wad of hot cotton wool that had been soaked in saline. He went on to finish the operation rapidly and nervously. When the drapes were removed, he was surprised to see Ruth looking up at him and smiling. She spoke quietly, "Well, little brother, have you finished? I knew you could do it."

Penfield went to the dressing room to change out of his scrubs and began crying. He was distraught. He felt he had failed. He almost lost his sister on the OR table, and he couldn't remove the entire tumor. He sat for a while talking to himself, wondering whether the large operation he performed on his sister's frontal lobe would alter her personality and turn her into a different person.

But Ruth was okay. She had only mild changes in her behavior. She made an excellent recovery, her headaches resolved, and her vision remained stable. Penfield sent her back to California by train with her mother. Ruth continued to thrive. On the first Monday after arriving home, her husband Jack took her to a dinner dance at the Rotary Club. She thought she might have ended up in a wheelchair after the surgery and was grateful and amazed that she could dance. The other attendees were equally surprised.

The pathology turned out to be an oligodendroglioma, a tumor of the supporting cells of the brain that make myelin, a substance that insulates the nerves. It was ironic that these supporting cells, the oligodendrocytes that turned neoplastic, were the very cells Penfield had studied while working with Hortega in Madrid. Penfield had looked at the tissue specimen under the microscope himself and thought the tumor had malignant features. He arranged for his sister to receive a series of X-ray treatments in LA to slow the growth of the tumor.

A year later, Ruth wrote her brother on December 11, 1929, the anniversary of the operation, "This has been the happiest year of my life."

Penfield wrote in his biography, "To the patient, I suppose, life that is granted unexpectedly must seem a priceless gift." Back in LA, Ruth remained well for two years. Then she developed a rapid return of symptoms, with severe progressive headaches and vomiting along with bulging of the scalp at her prior surgical site. It was clear that the tumor had recurred. This time, Penfield had her take a weeklong train ride to Boston, where he joined her to have Cushing do the repeat surgery.

Cushing operated on November 11, 1930, and debulked the tumor, writing rather bluntly in his operative note, "I was somewhat embarrassed by the position of the old bone flap," and made it larger. The tumor was again found to be an oligodendroglioma. Ruth had a slower recovery from surgery this time, but she stabilized. She returned to LA by train, where she did well initially and lived comfortably for six months before the tumor regrew explosively. She died with recurrent seizures and paralysis on her left side. Remarkably, four years later, in 1935, Penfield published his sister's case in the journal *Brain*, in which he described the subtle frontal lobe changes she developed after surgical resection of her tumor.

Penfield was grateful to Cushing for helping with his sister's case and wrote him a heartfelt note, "I want to thank you for all that you did for her. Simply to postpone death is very much worthwhile, for life when we measure it by weeks and months becomes a very precious thing."

Almost a century has passed since Penfield's courageous resection of his sister's brain tumor. Phenomenal advances in technology over the years have led to dramatic improvements in neurosurgical morbidity and mortality. My friend Stewie's life was prolonged for a time, and I hope his quality of life was meaningful. The toxicity of chemotherapy is substantial, though with modern targeted treatments there has been a considerable reduction in side effects. One thing that has never changed over time is the value we place on life and the importance of preserving it with quality. That value has remained timeless.

CHAPTER 18

Humility

"It ain't the heat, it's the humility."

Yogi Berra
Iconic American professional
baseball catcher and manager

The first time I met Liam Brown, he was not happy to see me. It was early in the morning on Saturday, October 21, 2023, and I was making rounds on the pediatric neurosurgery service at Johns Hopkins Hospital. Liam had been having headaches, and his mom, Mandy Bloodworth, had brought him to the Emergency Room the night before. He was a skinny little guy with a cute gap between his upper two front teeth. He was wearing a pair of slightly oversized glasses with black rims and had an iPad on his lap and his stuffed animal, a monkey, by his side. He had been kept NPO (Latin: *nil per os*, "nothing by mouth") by the ER for an MRI of the brain. The scanner was backed up, and Liam's study didn't get done until 2 a.m. He was exhausted. He had been up almost all night.

Liam gave me a glaring look and said, "It's not fair. I'm hungry, and I need to eat right now." I had seen the MRI before I came into his room and had already formulated a plan that didn't require him to be NPO for the day. So, I said, "Sure thing. Let's bring you some breakfast." He broke into a broad smile, and we bonded instantly.

Liam had been a healthy seven-year-old right-handed boy with a history of an attention-deficit disorder, for which he took medication. He was in school in the first grade, where he was an excellent student. Three weeks earlier, he started to complain of intermittent diffuse headaches, sometimes accompanied by vomiting. The headaches were often in the morning but could come on any time of day. Initially, Mandy thought they were due to allergies.

The headaches continued and worsened. Then on Wednesday, October 18, Liam began to complain of double vision. His schoolteacher noticed that his left eye was turned inward. She pointed it out to his mother, who agreed. Mandy brought Liam to see Dr. Paul Lomonico, his pediatrician, who ordered a non-contrast MRI of his brain. The MRI was performed on Friday, October 20, at an imaging center in Owings Mills, MD. After the scan, Mandy had left to drive Liam to their home in Bel Air, Maryland, and was on the road when she got a call from the radiologist.

"We didn't realize that you left," he said. "I'm sorry to tell you this, but your child has a very large brain tumor. I want you to go directly to the Johns Hopkins Emergency Room. We made a call. They are expecting you."

Mandy went into a state of shock. She was driving on Falls Road when she got the call, and the road had no shoulder. She immediately turned onto Greenspring Valley Road, where there was a shoulder, stopped the car, and got out to make phone calls to her family. I know the area well because I live nearby. Mandy was petrified and wanted to share the news without having to break down crying in front of Liam. She completed the calls and then nervously made the half-hour drive to the Hopkins ER, where she and Liam would end up spending the night. Shortly after arriving, she was joined by her close-knit family, which included her wife Christina, her ex-husband Darrell Brown, his wife Kayla, and her parents.

The doctors reviewed the scan, confirmed the finding of a brain tumor, and ordered a contrast-enhanced MRI to better define it. That was the study that couldn't be performed until 2 a.m. Mandy's family waited with them until Liam went off for the MRI and then left. Mandy and her ex-husband stayed with Liam in the ER through a sleepless night.

So, it was early on that Saturday morning that I first met Liam and his exhausted parents. I immediately became his new best friend because I allowed him to eat. I went on to examine him and found that he had papilledema (swelling of the optic discs) and a left esotropia (eye turned inward) due to pressure on the abducens cranial nerve, whose function is to turn the eye outward). These findings confirmed that Liam's headache was due to increased intracranial pressure.

The MRI demonstrated that the increased pressure was due to a large brain tumor in the right parietal lobe. It is interesting that the left abducens palsy was on the side opposite his tumor. The reason for that is the nerve palsy was not caused by direct compression from the tumor, but rather from indirect diffuse increased pressure inside the skull. The abducens nerve has the longest intracranial course of all the cranial nerves and is sensitive to pressure. Thus, an abducens nerve palsy can be a false localizing sign if one uses it to determine the side of a mass in the brain. But one cause for an abducens palsy, as was the case for Liam, is increased pressure from a brain tumor.

The MRI showed a large lobulated cystic and solid brain tumor in the right parietal lobe that enhanced avidly after the administration of intravenous contrast. There was significant edema surrounding the tumor that caused mass effect with pressure on the brain.

I reviewed the images with Mandy and Darrell, and we admitted Liam to the PICU, where he was placed on dexamethasone, a steroid, to reduce brain swelling, and levetiracetam, a medication to prevent seizures. By the next day, Liam's headache had improved, as had his abducens nerve palsy. The tumor was large, and we wanted to give time for the steroids to kick in and reduce the brain swelling. We made a plan for surgery the following day, Monday, October 23.

Early on Monday morning, Mandy, with her entire family at the bedside, said a quick goodbye to Liam as he was whisked off to the OR for surgery. Things had happened so quickly that Mandy was still in a state of shock and hadn't really had enough time to fully comprehend what was going on. It helped that Liam was engrossed in his iPad and didn't even look up to say goodbye. He was handling things better than his family, who stood silently in his room, each member aware that he was about to undergo a serious operation on his brain.

In the OR, we got Liam asleep, positioned him with his right side up, and registered him to the computer-based image guidance system to help us find the safest trajectory to the tumor. I was working with a superb team—our fellow, Rachel Pruitt, and resident, James Feghali. We performed the craniotomy, opened the dura, and found the tumor with the help of image guidance and ultrasonography. It was located about 1.5 centimeters below the surface of the brain. The brain was under pressure from the tumor and the surrounding edema and began to herniate out of the skull. The anesthesia team took measures to help relax the brain, and we began to remove the mass under the guidance of our operating microscope.

There were two things that made Liam's surgery a little tricky. First, the tumor was located just off midline, directly underneath the superior anastomotic vein of Trolard, named after the nineteenth-century French anatomist, Jean Baptiste Paulin Trolard. Trolard described the blood vessel that bears his name in his doctoral thesis in 1868, working in Algeria at the Algiers Preparatory College of Medicine. It is a large essential vein that drains blood from the cerebral hemisphere into the large midline superior sagittal sinus and ultimately back to the heart. We had to work carefully with microdissection to avoid injuring the vein, which could cause cerebral venous infarction, or stroke.

The second concern was that the tumor was in a portion of the parietal (sensory) lobe of the brain that sits directly behind and intimately adjacent to the primary motor cortex, which controls movement on the contralateral side of the body. To protect the motor cortex from injury, we used neurophysiologic monitoring, placing a phase-reversal electrode on the surface of the brain to help us identify and stay clear of the motor cortex.

The tumor was somewhat firm and had a surprisingly good plane that allowed us to separate it from the surrounding brain. The frozen section showed a primary tumor of the brain. We were able to achieve a gross total removal, and we put Liam's head back together. I was feeling pretty good when I went to talk to Liam's family.

The surgery took six hours. There was a lot of nervous energy in the waiting room. Mandy was still overcome by fright. The rest of the family had been there with her the entire time, fretful, struggling to distract themselves by pacing and trying to eat, even though they weren't hungry.

"Well, we were able to get the tumor out," I said, smiling and hoping to help reduce the tension. "The brain was under pressure, but we found a good plane around it, and it looks as if we were able to remove the entire thing. We'll have to wait a few days for the final diagnosis, but I think it might be a low-grade glioma, which would be a good thing. The breathing tube is out, and Liam is starting to wake up. You'll be able to see him in the PICU in a few minutes."

The anxiety level in the room came down quickly. We walked over to see Liam in the PICU. He was wide awake but was feisty and emotional. "Where's my iPad?" he asked. The family was overjoyed that their Liam was back. And I was relieved to see him moving his limbs and playing video games. We had been able to remove the tumor using a "lazy S" incision on the right side of his scalp. Liam had asked for a Mohawk haircut before the operation, so we gave him one. We also placed a turban bandage on his head in the shape of his precious stuffed animal monkey. And to come full circle, we had placed a turban on his stuffed monkey, too, letting them both recover together.

Liam made a rapid recovery and was discharged home after a short hospital stay. His headache, papilledema, and double vision resolved, and his MRI confirmed gross total resection of the tumor. We sent him happily on his way with his iPad, stuffed monkey, and funky mohawk. We tapered him off his steroid medication and maintained him on levetiracetam prophylactically for a few more weeks to prevent seizures.

But in thinking about things later, I realized the mistake I had made. I should have been more careful with my words when I spoke to the family in the waiting room. To offer a bit of hope, I told them that I thought the tumor might be a low-grade glioma. That's what I believed based on my intraoperative findings. The problem is that I didn't know the final diagnosis at the time I spoke to the family. Although everything I told them was true, I shouldn't have provided them with an opportunity for false hope. I should have waited for the final diagnosis to come back before offering my personal prognostication.

As it turned out, my guess about the diagnosis was wrong. The pathologic diagnosis returned supratentorial ependymoma, ZFTA-fusion positive, with homozygous deletion of CDKN2A, WHO grade 3 with sarcomatous changes. That's a mouthful. The main takeaway is that it was a malignant tumor. Brain cancer. Liam would require postoperative radiation therapy. Ependymomas are the third most common brain tumors of childhood, after gliomas and medulloblastomas. The alphabet soup in the name describes molecular markers that may prove helpful in directing further treatment strategies.

The diagnosis of a brain tumor in a child is a traumatic event for everyone involved and often places painful strains on the entire family. Although Liam's diagnosis was harrowing and heartbreaking, it helped bring his blended family even closer together. Just before he began radiation therapy, the whole clan got together for a Thanksgiving dinner. They were filled with hope.

Liam received outpatient proton beam radiation therapy under the direction of Dr. Sahaja Acharya at the Johns Hopkins Sibley Memorial Hospital in Washington, DC. Treatments were given five days a week over seven weeks. Liam was a tough little guy and went through each of the daily sessions without sedation. The treatments began in November and finished in January. Liam stayed in a hotel room with Mandy during the weekdays and went home for weekends. It wasn't fun going through radiation therapy over the Christmas holiday, but Liam and Mandy decorated the hotel room and got a tree to make things seem a little more cheerful.

After a long slog, Liam finally finished his cancer treatments on January 25, 2024. It was an emotional day, with about twenty family members present, each wearing a "Relative of a Warrior" T-shirt or sweatshirt. The event was streamed to his entire first-grade class, who celebrated with him. He returned to school and was back to his old self throughout the next year.

In October 2024, out of the blue, Liam developed the sudden onset of headache and vomiting. Workup with MRI showed a new right parietal brain tumor just medial to the site of the tumor we removed a year ago. It must have grown very quickly because an MRI performed two months earlier showed no evidence of tumor.

So, a year after his initial tumor resection, we went back to the OR on November 7, 2024, and removed the new tumor. This time, I worked with Kurt Lehner, our gifted chief resident, who was soon to become our pediatric neurosurgery fellow. The surgery was tricky because the tumor was adherent to the superior sagittal sinus, the large venous pipe that drains blood from the brain back to the heart. Fortunately, we were able to tease the tumor off the sinus and get a gross total removal.

Liam bounced back nicely and was watching videos on his iPad the morning after his surgery. Pathology was the same as it was a year earlier, a relapse of the aggressive malignant tumor, ependymoma with sarcomatous change. This time, Liam was treated by Dr. Michael Koldobskiy of oncology with six monthly intravenous cycles of ICE chemotherapy. Mike is a compassionate physician whose patients call him Dr. K because his last name is a tongue-twister to pronounce. ICE is a high-powered regimen consisting of ifosfamide, carboplatin, and etoposide. It wasn't an easy time for Liam, who had to be hospitalized from time to time for fevers due to chemotherapy-induced pancytopenia (low blood counts), but he held his ground, bounced back quickly, and returned to grade school, which he truly loves.

Liam is now off all medication and is happy that his hair has grown back. He is in remission, and his MRI shows no evidence of tumor. He is nine years old, in the third grade, functioning above his grade level, and reading *Harry Potter* books to the younger kids on the school bus. He enjoys playing baseball and particularly likes to play video games with his friends on Roblox. He is being followed closely with surveillance MRIs. He wants to be a YouTuber when he grows up.

Battling pediatric brain cancer is no walk in the park and takes a toll on the patient, family, and all health-care givers involved. We are delighted that Liam is in remission, and as we face the unknown, we hope it will last forever.

I am still humbled by the mistake I made early on, jumping the gun in the OR waiting room and sharing my thought that the tumor might have been low-grade, which it was not. In trying to offer hope, I had unintentionally introduced false hope. It is not always easy to find the proper balance between honesty and hope. If we had gone in thinking the tumor was malignant and later learned it was benign, a mistake like the one I made could be forgiven. It's much harder for a family to believe that the tumor is benign, only to find out later that it's malignant.

I've been humbled in my career more times than I wish to remember. I can't say I've ever enjoyed the experience, but it has always led to something positive, offering me an opportunity for self-improvement.

Humility is a critical component in the art of healing. The word is derived from the Latin *humilis*, the act of being humble. Humility is the antithesis of arrogance. It is not a weakness. It is not indecisiveness. It is not courtesy. Humility is the virtuous quality of having a modest assessment of one's own importance, of having an accurate understanding of self-worth. It is the ability to embrace and accept weakness. Humility can lead to strength. It can lead to personal growth. I have often learned more from failure than from success.

On May 1, 1889, William Osler coined the term Aequanimitas as the title of his valedictory address to new medical students on his leaving the University of Pennsylvania to become the first physician-in-chief at Johns Hopkins. He believed Aequanimitas to be the principal quality of the good physician. He considered Aequanimitas (Latin: *aequo animo*, "with even mind") equivalent to equanimity, "coolness and presence of mind under all circumstances." Equanimity is composure, mental calmness amid storm, clearness of temper even in moments of great peril.

Humility is an essential part of equanimity and has an important role in healing. To Osler, the grace of humility was a precious gift. He believed that recognition of our own fallibility would help us sympathize with the mistakes of others. Osler emphasized the importance of balancing head with heart for the physician. The great physician and surgeon must practice with both. C. S. Lewis, the British writer and literary scholar, said, "Humility is not thinking less of yourself, it's thinking of yourself less." Humility is the component of healing that comes from the heart.

Thinking of yourself less sometimes means allowing yourself to become more vulnerable. Vulnerability is a type of humility. Vulnerability is not weakness; it's actually a form of strength. In the words of the contemporary American poet and philosopher Criss Jami, "To share your weakness is to make yourself vulnerable. To make yourself vulnerable is to show your strength."

Vulnerability sometimes means letting your guard down. Vulnerability can make one appear more human. For the treating physician, it can have a powerful effect, helping to strengthen the all-important bond between doctor and patient. It can be effective in helping physicians earn the trust of patients and families. This is particularly important for physicians like me who care for children who have been stricken with serious illness.

At the risk of personal embarrassment, I will share a story about the role humility played in shaping my own development.

In the 1970s, I was a medical student in New York City at Cornell University Medical College/New York Hospital. To maintain my sanity and take a break from the endless hours of rote memorization of Latin and Greek terms for medical disorders, I decided on a whim to take up the art of sleight of hand. It provided me with a nice distraction from the daily grind. And it gave me an opportunity to entertain my friends and colleagues as I improved my technique with practice. I used to carry a medical bag with me when I was on the wards in the hospital. It was filled with an assortment of non-medical things like sponge balls, coins, silk scarves, and decks of cards. I had a lot of fun with this hobby, and I would often entertain my young patients on the pediatric wards by making things disappear in front of their eyes.

At the time, I was fortunate to have the opportunity to do a mini apprenticeship with a world-class magician. He called himself *The Great Slydini.* Humility may not have been his strong suit, but he had exceptional manual dexterity and was an unparalleled master of misdirection. I'd heard about him from a friend. Whenever I had the opportunity, I would sneak away to take lessons in close-up prestidigitation from the guru himself in his small office on West Forty-Fifth Street.

His professional name was Tony Slydini, but his given name at birth in Foggia, Italy, had been Quintino Marucci. When he came to New York in the 1930s, his fellow magician friends felt he needed a more appropriate stage name. *Tony* was short for Quintino, *Sly* was because he was a shrewd performer, and *dini* was an attempt to link him to the grandmaster, Harry Houdini. Tony Slydini had arrived.

When I studied with him, he was elderly, somewhat frail, and at the twilight of his career. He was an unassuming man who spoke slowly with a very thick accent. At times, I found myself mimicking his behavior, speaking slowly to him, thinking, incorrectly, that he might be having trouble processing everything I was saying. I was wrong. No words were necessary for his art. He was a genius. He had gifted hands that could make things disappear right before your eyes. It was mind-boggling, and I was hooked.

As an amateur magician, I found myself one sunny Sunday afternoon going for a walk in Washington Square Park in the Greenwich Village neighborhood of Lower Manhattan. The park, named for George Washington, is one of the jewels of the city. While I was there, I stumbled on a crowd of people who were standing in a circle near the celebrated marble Washington Arch, watching the work of another renowned master magician. His name was Philippe Petit, and he was a French street performer and high-wire artist. He had recently gained international fame on the morning of August 7, 1974, when he executed an unauthorized walk across a tightrope he had strung between the twin towers of the World Trade Center in New York City.

Somehow, he had managed to rig a 450-pound cable between the twin towers, over 1,300 feet in the air. He spent forty-five minutes on the high wire—walking, dancing, lying down, and bowing to the spectators below. At the completion of his performance, he was promptly arrested by the New York City Police Department and forced to undergo a psychiatric evaluation. Charges were ultimately dropped, however, when he agreed to perform pro bono for a group of young children.

When I met him in Washington Square Park, Petit was dressed in all black, juggling three clubs while walking across a tightrope that he had strung between two trees. Then he jumped off the rope and began riding a unicycle rapidly around a large circle he had outlined. There must have been a hundred people lined up around the circle watching the performance. Suddenly, he stopped riding and jumped off his unicycle right in front of me. He began juggling three balls, looking directly at me. He was a mime artist—there was no talking. I don't have any idea what caused him to approach me, but I knew nothing good was going to come of this, so I kept looking down at the ground, trying not to make eye contact.

Then he put one ball down and began juggling two balls with one hand, eliciting a round of applause from his rapt audience. Juggling the two balls in one hand, he then offered them to me, beckoning me to do the same. He did this three times, and each time, I shook my head no and stepped back. I felt that I was a pretty street-smart guy, and I was certain that he was up to something that would end up leaving me totally embarrassed. There was no way I was going to let that happen.

But Petit wouldn't stop. I must have looked like an easy mark to him. He began to stir up the audience enthusiastically, and they all started applauding and yelling and egging me on as he continued gesturing for me to take the two balls and juggle. At this point, I thought, I could resist no longer. I felt pretty confident at the time because I knew something that he didn't know. In addition to being an amateur magician, I was also an amateur juggler. In fact, I was a card-carrying member of the IJA, the International Jugglers' Association. Two balls in one hand? No big deal. That was Introductory Juggling. Juggling 101. The basics. I could do that in my sleep. What could go wrong?

The next thing I knew, Petit had pulled me into the center of the ring. He took my left arm and moved it behind my back, at the same time placing the two balls in my right hand. Then he stood back and watched with astonishment as I casually and flawlessly juggled the two balls with one hand. The audience went wild with raucous applause. Feeling proud of myself, I took several bows. I even felt a little sorry for Petit. He'd picked on the wrong guy, and I had spoiled his act. Or so I believed. He appeared stunned and quickly ushered me back to my place with the rest of the spectators, where I took a final bow.

And then the hammer dropped, and it hit hard. Petit ran back to the center of the arena and held up my wristwatch, along with its leather strap that had previously been tightly fastened around my wrist, for all to see.

He had distracted me with the juggling and was able to take the watch and band completely off my left wrist in the span of about one second, without me, or anyone else, noticing anything. I felt humiliated and turned beet red. I wanted to crawl under a rock and hide. The crowd roared, laughing louder than ever. I had been duped by the master. How could I have been so naïve as to make a fool of myself by taking multiple bows just for juggling two balls? What was I thinking?

In the end, it was all in good fun, though I did make sure I got my watch back. This Philippe Petit was a real pro in the art of distraction. He had an incredibly light touch and could easily have had a career as a pickpocket. That day, I learned another valuable lesson about humility and the importance of not taking oneself too seriously. And I will never again trust a mime dressed in all black riding a unicycle.

So, these are some thoughts about the role of humility in my personal life and in the practice of medicine. The good physician understands the patient's disease and focuses on treating the disorder. The humble physician tries to understand what it feels like to have the disease and concentrates more on healing the patient. The humble physician is less self-centered and more focused on the patient, on expressing empathy and compassion.

It is wise to recognize that even the greatest clinicians have limits to their abilities. Humility is an attribute that enables individuals to recognize their true place in the overall scheme of things. That can sometimes be a hard pill to swallow. It is also important to note that, at some point in life, the doctor becomes the patient. It is inevitable. In this sense, there is little that separates the most commanding and authoritative healers from those who have been under their care. Disease is a great equalizer. Humility serves to take physicians down a notch, reminding us of our own insignificance and helping us focus on delivering the finest patient-centered care possible.

Let me end as I began, with the wise words of Moses Maimonides from almost a thousand years ago, "May I never forget that the patient is a fellow creature in pain. May I never consider him merely a vessel of disease." These words still ring true.

Today, we practice medicine much differently than Maimonides did back in the Middle Ages. We work with sophisticated minimally invasive surgical tools, including MRI-guided deep brain stimulation, high-intensity focused ultrasound (HIFU), and laser interstitial thermal therapy (LITT). These are devices that Maimonides could never have dreamed of having. Such major advances in technology are of great value to modern physicians treating the diseases we encounter.

But restoring the patient to health requires more. It requires the softer, humanistic elements of patient care as well. In the art of healing, technology and humanity are synergistic. Technology treats the disease; humanity heals the patient.

Humility is a component of humanity; humility is an act of kindness. Those who practice humility do so without the expectation of anything in return. Kindness is a simple but powerful component of the art of healing. It enables the heart to rule the head. It has many positive physiological effects. It also increases connectivity, thereby strengthening the essential doctor-patient bond. As the Greek fabulist Aesop noted, "No act of kindness, no matter how small, is wasted."

Kindness goes a long way.

APPENDIX: WHERE ARE THEY NOW? (LISTED CHRONOLOGICALLY)

Christopher L. Taylor, MD
Associate Professor and Vice Chair of Neurosurgery
University of New Mexico, Albuquerque, New Mexico

Jesse L. Winer, MD
Associate Professor of Neurosurgery
Doernbecher Children's Hospital Oregon Health and Science University, Portland, Oregon

Jeremy Amps, MD
Attending Neurosurgeon
Cleveland Clinic, Cleveland, Ohio

Jonathan P. Miller, MD
Professor and Chair of Neurosurgery
SUNY Upstate Medical University, Syracuse, New York

Tina C. Rodrigue, MD
Private Practice Neurosurgeon
Sentara CarePlex Hospital, Hampton, Virginia

Ali Najafi, MD
Private Practice, Minimally Invasive Spine Surgery
Fresno, California

Scellig S.D. Stone, MD, PhD
Associate Professor of Neurosurgery, Director of Stereotactic and Functional Neurosurgery, Co-Director of Epilepsy Center
Boston Children's Hospital, Harvard Medical School

Bradley Gross, MD
Associate Professor of Neurosurgery,
Director of Endovascular Surgery
University of Pittsburgh Medical Center

Shekar Kurpad, MD, PhD
Professor of Neurosurgery, Director, Institute of Neurosciences
Medical College of Wisconsin, Milwaukee, Wisconsin

Rachel M. Pruitt, MD
Assistant Professor of Neurosurgery; Attending Pediatric Neurosurgeon, Cohen Children's Hospital
Zucker School of Medicine/Hofstra/Northwell Medical Center, New Hyde Park, New York

Connor Liu, MD
Senior Neurosurgery Resident
Johns Hopkins University School of Medicine, Baltimore, Maryland

Andrew J. Kobets, MD
Assistant Professor of Neurosurgery; Attending Pediatric Neurosurgeon, Children's Hospital at Montefiore
Albert Einstein College of Medicine, Bronx, New York

Risheng Xu, MD, PhD
Associate Professor of Neurosurgery;
Assistant Director, Neurosurgery Residency Program
Johns Hopkins University School of Medicine, Baltimore, Maryland

Jignesh Tailor, MD, PhD
Assistant Professor of Neurosurgery
Riley Children's Health, Indiana University School of Medicine

Andreas C. Tomac, MD, PhD
Private Practice Neurosurgeon
Fort Lauderdale, Florida

Tej Azad, MD
Neurosurgical Spine Fellow
Johns Hopkins University School of Medicine, Baltimore, Maryland

Baha Muhsen, MD
Consultant Neurosurgeon
King Hussein Cancer Center, Amman, Jordan

Adam Ammar, MD
Private Practice Pediatric Neurosurgeon
New Jersey Pediatric Neuroscience
Institute, Morristown, New Jersey

Jawad Khalifeh, MD
Chief Resident in Neurosurgery
Johns Hopkins University School of
Medicine, Baltimore, Maryland

Shakeel A. Chowdhry, MD
Private Practice Neurosurgeon
Northshore Neurological Institute, Evanston, Illinois

Kurt Lehner, MD
Pediatric Neurosurgery Fellow
Johns Hopkins University School of
Medicine, Baltimore, Maryland

James Feghali, MD
Senior Neurosurgery Resident
Johns Hopkins University School of
Medicine, Baltimore, Maryland

ACKNOWLEDGMENTS

"The man who forgets to be thankful has fallen asleep in life."

ROBERT LOUIS STEVENSON

This book would not have been possible without the generous support of friends, colleagues, and family. I am deeply grateful to them for their time, thoughtfulness, and guidance.

To Dody Robinson, MD, my wife, for her perpetual calm demeanor, patience, and numerous insightful suggestions.

To Nate Cohen, MD, and Jeremy Cohen, my sons, and Emily Garvin, my daughter-in-law, for their tough love and critical editorial revisions.

To my oldest friend, Karen Endicott, for translating the book into English, even though that's my native language.

To Lynn Powell, award-winning author of *Framing Innocence*, for her mentorship and for teaching me restraint in the use of adverbs.

To Dan Stinebring, PhD, the smartest astrophysicist on the planet, for helping me make the stories come alive.

To my dear friend, Richa Mishra, MD, for her countless methodical reads and rereads to help me clean up the scientific jargon.

To Greg Johnson, my literary agent, for keeping me focused, organized, and motivated.

To the phenomenal staff at Post Hill Press, who were a joy to work with, for bringing this project to life, particularly: Lauren Campbell, managing editor; Debra Englander, consulting editor; and Brynlee Wolfe, production editor.

To Samantha Holmes, visual artist, for the striking author website she designed for me.

To the members of our weekly Pediatric Neuro-Oncology Conference at Johns Hopkins, particularly: Kenneth Cohen, MD, Eric Raabe, MD, PhD, Michael Koldobskiy, MD, PhD, Robyn Gartrell, MD, Jeffrey Rubens, MD, Sahaja Acharya, MD, Aylin Tekes, MD, Melike Guryildirim, MD, Doris Lin, MD, PhD, Charles Eberhart, MD, PhD, CJ Lucas, MD, Peter Burger, MD, and Neil Miller, MD, for their essential roles in the management of our shared patients.

To Jay Wellons, MD, MSPH, bestselling author of *All That Moves Us*, for his indispensable mentoring.

To David Sandberg, MD, bestselling author of *Brain and Heart*, for his extremely generous encouragement and wise counsel.

To Theodore Schwartz, MD, bestselling author of *Gray Matters*, for his continued support and judicious advice.

To my partners and physician assistants, Mari Groves, MD, Eric Jackson, MD, Dody Robinson, MD, Ed Ahn, MD, Stephanie Berry, PA-C, Kristin Jones, PA-C, Heather Kerber, PA-C, and Kelly Hartnett, PA-C, who provided unparallel care for many of the children I have written about here.

To the OR nurses, surgical technologists, anesthesiologists and intensivists at Johns Hopkins, Boston Children's, and Rainbow, the unsung heroes who work tirelessly to provide exceptional care to our patients.

To my amazingly dedicated and kind-hearted office staff at Johns Hopkins—Kim Patton, Shirley Simon, Tina Rybczynski, and Jaime Ryan—whose dedication and diligence have kept our busy clinical practice on track.

To my former extraordinary medical office supervisor at Rainbow Babies & Children's Hospital, Helen Novotney, who is featured in some of these stories.

To Henry Brem, MD, Chetan Bettegowda, MD, PhD, and my resident, fellow, and attending colleagues in the Johns Hopkins Department of Neurosurgery, the greatest partners in the greatest neurosurgery department in the world, for inspiring me to be a better doctor.

To Rachel Brem, MD, bestselling author of *No Longer Radical: Understanding Mastectomies And Choosing the Breast Cancer Care That's Right For You,* for her encouragement and for helping me navigate the complex world of publishing.

Finally, to my brave patients and their families, for allowing me to tell their powerful and poignant stories.